The Home Chef's Kitchen Medical Emergency Guide

The Home Chef's Kitchen Medical Emergency Guide

Jack Sholl

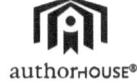

authorHOUSE®

AuthorHouse™
1663 Liberty Drive
Bloomington, IN 47403
www.authorhouse.com
Phone: 1-800-839-8640

Published by AuthorHouse   02/01/2013

ISBN: 978-1-4772-8863-4 (sc)
ISBN: 978-1-4772-8862-7 (hc)
ISBN: 978-1-4772-8864-1 (e)

This book is printed on acid-free paper.

Contents

Introduction

Ever since man, foraging for food in the jungle, received his first concussion from a falling coconut, the kitchen has been a potentially dangerous place.

Today, we don't have to climb trees to obtain a savory meal. The 21st-century home kitchen contains all the ingredients necessary to produce a meal that rivals the best of haute cuisine restaurants. As a result of the dining craze of the past decade and a great global economy, more and more home chefs are transferring the culinary delights of the four-star restaurant to their home dining rooms.

Yet despite the many technological wonders of the modern kitchen and the constant striving of appliance manufacturers to improve and build in safety measures, the kitchen, in many respects, remains what it has always been: a potentially dangerous place. Most superb dishes usually require dicing, slicing, heating, boiling or cutting, all time-honored methods of fine food preparation. Yet, whether they be done automatically or by hand, each action presents the potential opportunity for self-injury or injury to a guest.

Even eating the simplest food can be hazardous. Just ask George W. Bush.

Yes, President Bush.

President Bush lost consciousness and fainted while eating a pretzel in the White House. And it wasn't a joke. The President was watching a televised National Football game and munching pretzels when one went astray. He fainted when his heart rate temporarily dropped after the swallowed pretzel got stuck in his throat. The President sustained an abrasion on his left cheek and a bruise on his lower lip when he fell over.

What happened?

A neurological exam pointed to vasovagal fainting. In such cases, the body sends a signal to the heart via the vagus nerve that slows the heart rate enough to cut off the oxygen supply and cause a fainting spell.

So, if it can happen with a mere pretzel to the President of the United States in the White House, there's no reason to think that the same couldn't happen with, for example, that tempting bowl of chef's nuts, almonds basted in sherry with a touch of chili pepper, deep fried camembert-filled samosas, a wad of sushi or dozens of other gourmet appetizers and dishes.

An estimated one-quarter of a million Americans are annually brought to hospital emergency rooms or clinics for injuries that occurred in the kitchen. Considering that many smaller injuries, a small burn, cut or sprain, never get to the emergency room, the number of kitchen and cooking injuries is no doubt much higher. And according to the U.S. Centers for Disease Control, over 200 diseases can be spread through food. Studies report that some 79 million food-borne illnesses occur the United States annually, resulting in 325,000 hospitalizations and 5,000 deaths.

This guide to kitchen emergencies is *not* intended to be all-inclusive for any emergency, because any type of emergency can happen in the kitchen, just as it can anywhere in the home or outside. It will instead suggest ways the practicing home chef can prepare an accident-free, worry-free and safe kitchen, and handle a number of medical emergencies and incidents that may occur. The suggestions herein are nothing new; they've been commonly and traditionally used by thousands of Boy Scouts, rescue workers, health workers, and military personnel, among others. The Chef's Home Kitchen Medical Emergency Guide brings together in one place those time-honored first-aid measures that apply to accidents that can, and often do, occur in the kitchen. The ultimate goal is to help ensure the home chef enjoy the joys of a well-cooked meal and a memorable, hassle-free dining experience.

At the outset, it must be emphasized that there is no—NOT ANY—substitute for prompt professional medical care in the event of a kitchen emergency. The guiding principle is that in the event of a kitchen medical emergency, the chef, sous chef, guests and others *immediately* dial 9-1-1 for paramedics, the fire department, police or any other emergency ambulance service, or be taken to the nearest emergency room or medical clinic, where professional medical advice and treatment can be secured. The home chef should have on hand a list of emergency facilities in his or her neighborhood, their telephone numbers and directions on how to get there. You will find in Chapter 15 a form used for listing the emergency facilities and services in your neighborhood. The home chef should tear this page from this book, fill in the telephone numbers and paste the sheet somewhere in the kitchen within easy access near the telephone. Chapter 15 also provides a simple blank map the home chef should also complete and post in the kitchen, as is often the case with these emergencies, the thought comes too late that the home chef doesn't have a clue as to where the nearest hospital or emergency medical facility is from his or her home. Emergency telephone numbers are also important to have immediately on hand because medical advice or rescue can be obtained by phone. Additionally, the home chef should consider a practice dry run to the emergency room.

While no one expects accidents, the very nature of an accident is unpredictable. Thus, prevention is the best guide. This book does not replace sound professional medical advice, but from a common sense standpoint gives practical and time-honored ways to help cope with a medical emergency in the kitchen.

Part of being a great chef is to operate a safe kitchen and dining establishment. All great restaurants, whether they be in hotels or elsewhere, provide first-aid training to chefs. In fact, first-aid training is part of the curriculum at all culinary schools. The home chef in his or her kitchen is in no different a situation. He or she should be likewise prepared for accidents and medical emergencies.

Bon appetite and safe cooking!

I

Cuts, Punctures, Lacerations and Bruises

Not long ago, Dr. P. invited us to Saturday-night dinner at his two-story, brick Tudor home in the hills overlooking the beautiful, rolling vineyards of Napa Valley. A prominent plastic surgeon by day and a gourmet chef of incomparable excellence by night, the dish he'd selected was the recipe of the year as selected by *Bon Appetite* magazine: cod fish over mashed potatoes. The idea was to use this variation of a simple-but-elegant, traditional French peasant meal to set off a sterling 1982 Cakebread Chardonnay, which had just reached its anticipated height of fermentation.

Needless say, the meal was exceptional and the wine outstanding. But we noticed as Dr. P. ladled the sauce beurre over the cod, that his fingers were bandaged. "Bad day in the operating room?" we inquired. "No," Dr. P. answered to our surprise, "bad day in the kitchen."

The situation was such: Dr. P. had left a two-pound fillet of frozen cod, flash-frozen in the Pacific Ocean but 24 hours earlier, in the refrigerator to thaw. When the moment came to begin the meal preparation, Dr. P. removed the fillet from the fridge, unwrapped it and washed it under cold water in the sink. The cod felt a little cold to the touch, so Dr. P., holding the fillet in his right hand, firmly prodded the white flesh of the cod with a fork. The result was unexpected and something that had never happened to him in twenty-five years of surgical practice in the operating room; the fork sailed through the cod fillet, went right through Dr. P.'s hand and pierced it with five-pointed prongs.

As a physician, Dr. P. knew that wounds to the to the epidermal layer of the skin can range from minor (a scratch) to severe (deep). In this instance, Dr. P. watched five little red circles of blood form on each of the inside fingers of his right hand.

Diagnosing the injury, Dr. P. first ran his hand under cold tap water and cleansed the wounds with soap. The second step was to staunch the blood flow with gauze, plentiful in the operating room, but absent in the kitchen. Thus, a towel sufficed for the moment.

Dr. P., again, from his operating room experience, knew it was important to put an antiseptic and antibiotic on these small punctures. To prevent infection in his own system, but equally important in this day and age, to insure that no-blood-borne viruses he may have encountered spread to any of the food he was working with. While he'd been tested for hepatitis, HIV and other similar infectious pathogens, he was quite familiar with the transmission routes of these diseases. He surely didn't want to take the chance that his guests would leave with more than memories of a good meal after they departed thanks to carelessness on his part.

As the leeks in the oven reached their point of perfection before burning, Dr. P. had to race to the bathroom medicine cabinet for adhesive bandages and an antiseptic. Then it was back to the kitchen to continue to stir the leeks, just in time.

What happened here illustrates what can happen to anyone while making any of hundreds of different meats, fish, fowl and other preparations. And if it can happen to a skilled surgeon of long practice, it can happen to the home gourmet chef who may have just raced home from the office to prepare or finish the evening dinner for family and friends.

Prodding a cod fillet with a pointy-pronged fork or knife while holding it in one's hand somehow becomes normal in the thrill of working in the gourmet kitchen—something neither an experienced surgeon or outdoorsman would do in normal context. Yet it is but one of a hundreds of different similar skin injuries that can happen in the kitchen when handling sharp cutlery.

Most of us can probably also relate when we hear of hands or fingers being pierced while placing lamb and onion chunks on a barbecue skewers or while inserting sharp pointed bamboo sticks into a sushi roll; of cases where hands punching aeration holes in aluminum foil-wrapped baked potatoes were pierced; of slicing a finger of the edge of a sharp can lid while opening a can, or impaling a hand on a submerged knife caught upright in the sink's garbage disposal. Likewise, the nipped or sliced finger while shaving or paring a small vegetable or fruit, like a kiwi, is all too well known. The upshot can range from a small scratch or drop of blood to deep lacerations of veins or striking a nerve (as in acupuncture) and causing paralysis or neurological damage.

How much easier would it have been if the antiseptic, gauze and adhesive bandages were in a handy first aid kit in a kitchen cabinet, so that a minor accident could be repaired without needlessly wasting time searching for first-aid items? (Chapter 14.) Besides the obvious medical implications, five minutes solving a small and important emergency of this type could make the difference between a good meal and a great a meal, for example, as the heat on the range may need to be lowered or turned off, to stop sauces and reductions from congealing and/or depriving vegetables or meats of perfect flavor.

While not exhaustive, here are the main types of cuts, lacerations and bruises that can potentially occur in the kitchen accidentally while one is distracted, or unclear about the techniques of using sharp instruments. Again, nothing can replace proper medical care from a qualified medical practitioner, and professional medical treatment should always be sought.

Deep puncture wounds

Deep puncture wounds—such as from a knife, skewer or wine corkscrew—are typically longer than one inch deep. They are also characterized by inability to stop the bleeding.

In the case of a severe puncture wound, the guiding principle is to dial 9-1-1 or go *immediately* to an emergency room or doctor.

Ideally, use a piece of thick sterilized gauze to press on the wound. In the event clean gauze isn't available, use any cloth, the cleanest available, to press on the wound. In the kitchen, this could include towels, dishrags or napkins. Failing to find any of these, remove and use your shirt, socks or another clean clothing item. If none of these are possibilities, use your hand, pressing the palm firmly over the wound. It's always important to remember that whatever you use to staunch the wound, cleanliness of the material is necessary to prevent later infection.

It's also important to remember not to press directly on any object that might be stuck or impaled in the wound. Instead press around it. This is particularly important with eye injuries or broken bones. And never try to remove something firmly stuck in a wound. Leave that to the doctor. In the event of a bleeding eye wound, cover the eyes lightly (never put direct pressure on an eye wound) with gauze or bandages, and head for the emergency room on the double.

When the bleeding stops, the cloth being used should not be removed. Leave it in place and use more cloths to cover it.

If the bleeding won't stop after several—say five—minutes, find an artery and apply pressure with your thumb. Points that an artery can be found are in the neck, elbow (inside), wrist (inside), groin, knee (back) and top of the feet.

You may also wish to use a tourniquet to stop severe bleeding. The tourniquet should be applied above the wound toward the heart, so the blood flow from the heart to the wound is restricted. However, you must loosen the tourniquet periodically to prevent gangrene from setting in. A simple tourniquet can be made from a strip of cloth wound on the limb (above the wound) and drawn tight by twisting the end of the cloth with a stick or even a flat-edged dinner knife from the table. Rubber tourniquets can be purchased, and the chef may consider keeping one in his or her kitchen medicine chest. Also, placing the injured limb higher than the heart can reduce the flow of blood.

Nerve damage

Sharp pointed objects, such as many found in the home kitchen, are also capable of striking nerves. The result can be temporary paralysis of a limb, or worse, some form of permanent damage to the nervous system.

In the kitchen, fish, meats and even some vegetables could potentially pose this harm if not handled properly and carefully. Take as an example the rockfish, as commonly found in supermarkets as red snapper, or the catfish or puffer fish, which have bony spikes. Or any fish, for that matter, where the chef may be preparing or deboning a whole fish. A jab from a pointed, razor-sharp bone (much like a needle) can easily go through the skin and strike a nerve. Many a sole Meunière has had to be completed by a one-handed chef whose other hand was rendered inoperative by a fish-boned hand. And heaven help the right-handed chef who, with the added pressure of hosting, has got to work with only his or her left hand.

The best advice in the event of such an occurrence is to consult a neurologist if paralysis or numbness cannot be shaken off or if it doesn't dissipate.

Small cuts, wounds and bruises

Small cuts are characterized as generally being less than one-quarter inch deep and not too long.

Wash the wound with soap and water. Put an antiseptic or antibiotic on the cut or scrape to prevent infection. Then apply an adhesive bandage or similar bandage, such as a piece of gauze held by a surgical adhesive tape, or in a pinch, clear adhesive tape will suffice. Just remember not to apply the bandage so tightly that it stops the blood flowing to that area.

Remember that, as with any cut in or out of the kitchen, a cut from metal, particularly metal with rust on it, may require a tetanus shot.

Glass

Broken dishes, glasses and jars frequently occur in the home kitchen. And all present the opportunity for shards of glass to cut or get embedded in the chef's hand or finger.

Glass cuts should be treated as any other cut or puncture, with the following important exceptions:

Don't apply pressure on a glass cut. Do not press hard on gauze or cloth to staunch bleeding, nor apply a tight bandage to a glass cut. The reason being pieces of glass, even minute, may be in the wound and pressing down would further complicate matters. Minute pieces of glass will eventually work their way upward naturally and slough off.

If a glass shard is visible and can easily be removed with a tweezers (from the chef's kitchen medical emergency kit), then you may attempt to carefully remove it. Otherwise, embedded glass is best left alone for the moment. Trying to remove it could severely complicate matters by doing more damage to tissue, nerves and blood vessels. An immediate trip to the emergency room or an emergency medical facility is called for, in this case.

Should a glass sliver or shard get embedded in an eye, never, ever apply pressure to the eyeball. Get to the emergency room immediately, or dial 9-1-1.

And never eat food that's been contaminated by glass. Even if you think you've removed all the shards, tiny, miniscule pieces may still be buried in the food. A companion and I once observed a group of highly educated physicians and medical practitioners devour exquisite and expensive caviar with glass fragments taken from a broken caviar jar top rather than throw the delicate black fish eggs away. Better to be safe than sorry. As ingested glass fragments can cause internal bleeding and, potentially, perforations of the colon, among other horrors. As a rule of thumb, then, spit out or throw out any food that's come in contact with broken or shattered glass. It's not worth the potential danger.

Slicing off the tip of a finger

As ghastly as it may sound, the risk of slicing off the tip or more of a finger in the kitchen is always there, especially for the unwary, distracted, rushed or intoxicated chef. Just think of the many great recipes that require mincing, dicing or slicing of vegetables with large chopping knives or cleavers and you'll get the picture.

Needless to say, should a digit be chopped or sliced off, dial 9-1-1 and/or drop everything and get to the closest emergency room.

As a first aid step, the blood flow should be stanched with a thick, sterile gauze bandage, as would be done with a puncture wound.

Depending upon the size of the injury, steps should also be taken to preserve the severed finger. Put the fingertip in a plastic bag and put it in the freezer of your refrigerator. Or depending upon time, fill the bag with ice from the freezer, and take it with you to the emergency room.

Again, depending upon the size of the injury, it should be noted that small slices of skin should eventually regenerate themselves.

Bruises

Bruises can occur in any number of ways in the home kitchen. A popular activity known among home chefs is smashing his or her thumb from pounding meat or fowl with a meat hammer. And just imagine how many fingers a contemporary corkscrew has pinched?

The treatment for this easily-acquired wound is similar to small cuts. Simply wash the wound and apply an antiseptic. Additionally, ice or an ice pack (ice in a plastic bag or towel) may be placed on the bruise to alleviate pain and help reduce swelling.

Broken fingers should be treated as any broken bone (Chapter 3.)

Precautions and preventive measures

Most common kitchen injuries can be avoided by the chef simply being aware of what he or she is doing and taking proper preventive measures. We recall an ancient patron of a notable French restaurant in midtown Manhattan toppling down the stairs to the men's room, glass goblet of red wine (no doubt of good vintage) in hand, resulting in large pieces of glass in and blood gushing form his forehead.

So:

- Slice away from you, never towards you.
- Never have a knife-edge or blade pointed toward you, always away.
- Never poke anything you're holding in your hand with a sharp pointed utensil. If you're going to poke or impale anything, put it on the kitchen counter or a cutting board or plate. The same for slicing things such as cheese blocks.
- Always make sure your fingers are sufficiently away from the part or section that's being cut. And take your time, don't rush.
- Always use properly sized knives and utensils, and use them in the right manner. For example, do not use a large cleaver to whack off potato slices.
- Handle fish bones and spiny vegetables—such as the artichoke—with respect and care.
- Always stack knives and forks downside in the dish-washer, utensil drainer or sink drainer.
- Throw out any food that may have become contaminated with glass.

II

Burns and Scalds

Of all the injuries that take place in the kitchen, burns and scalds are the most common. That's because unless you're an Eskimo—on second thought, even then—most food preparations in the kitchen require the use of heat in its many forms in varying degrees. Deep-frying oils, red-hot baking racks, boiling waters and sauces, sizzling sauté oils and juices, hot pans and handles are just a few of the many objects that can inflict injury in the kitchen unless care is taken when working around them. Further, using millions of gallons of cooking oil, margarine and butter for frying each year, Americans, in particular, should be well informed on burns.

Any type of burn and scald, or multiple burns, can potentially occur in the kitchen accidentally, while one is distracted or unclear about what one is doing. Hands and digits are not the only appendages susceptible to burns or scalds in the home chefferie. The groin, feet and ankles, for example, present vulnerable targets from a hot soup missing the bowl as it's poured.

The face, hair and eyes are all vulnerable, from a furnace-hot blast in the face while peering into the oven or splatters from a sauté pan, to be frizzed or crisped.

Beards depending on their length, can be a particular hazard in the kitchen. A beard might set easily ablaze as the chef, for example, hangs too close to the saucepan to sniff a reduction sauce. (A variation of this is the beard gets caught in an electric mixer, automatic bread maker, or garbage disposal.) (Chapter 4.)

Nevertheless, the most and potentially serious common kitchen accident that can inflict a serious burn, in particular of the hands, are water burns. And not just from boiling water. Most often, painful burns occur when the chef turns on the hot water tap on the sink and puts his or her hand under it to test the temperature. In cases like this, the chef can expect blistering with a resultant uncosmetic look. And in even more serious cases, infection.

Other common burns of the hands and fingers can occur when one is removing pots from the stove. For example, the home chef may, with naked hands, attempt to remove a hot pot lid thinking it will take only a second to place on the counter. Not so: the chef may find, as is usually the case, that the lid needs to be maneuvered on the counter. Considering the top is burning hot, this predicament unfailingly leads to burnt fingers. And of course everyone's familiar, at least figuratively, with burning one's fingers from handling a hot potato.

Burns come in four degrees of seriousness, depending upon how deep the heat has burnt into the skin.

Types of burns

A first-degree burn is characterized as a burn that has burnt the top or outer layer of the skin (epidermis). It can be quite painful.

A second-degree burn is characterized as a burn that burns the top and inner layers of the skin (dermis). Burns of this nature are very painful, and they can often blister or swell the skin.

A third-degree burn is one that goes right through all the layers of the skin (hypodermis). It doesn't hurt because it usually burns the nerve ending of the tissue. The skin looks white or charred black.

A fourth-degree burn, the most serious, burns right down to any organs below the skin.

As has been suggested throughout this book, anything that appears to be a third- or fourth-degree burn requires immediate professional medical help. Dial 9-1-1 or immediately head for the nearest emergency room.

For smaller burns, take a clean towel or cloth and put it under cool water. Wring the towel out and gently cover the burn. The burn can also be placed under cool running water or placed in a bowl, depending upon where the burn is located. Pain should subside. Don't use water for very large and sizable areas that have been burnt. Use sterile gauze or a clean towel or cloth.

Placing the limb upon which the burn is located higher than the heart can reduce swelling.

Preventive measures

Because they tend to be plentiful in the kitchen, fatty substances like butter, margarine, or shortening, as well as ice are common substances home chefs are tempted to use for alleviating burn pain. The basic guideline, however, is don't do it. The same for petroleum jelly, lotions or other salves. Also, don't puncture any blisters that may have formed, and certainly do not use any type of adhesive bandage or sticky surgical tape close to the burnt area. If for any reason, a patch of clothing has melted into the burn, do not pull the material away. Put gauze or a clean towel or cloth over the spot as it is.

It's imperative that the home chef has a pair of good hot pads that fit the hands like a glove. Common hand burns are caused by a chef impetuously grabbing the handle of a pan or pot on the stove to make a sudden modification in the cooking process. Usually, because of the need for swiftness of the maneuver, hands are sacrificed for the sake of avoiding an overcooked dish.

It's important to remember that not all hot pads are the same. Some are nothing more than thick cloth that allow dangerous heat to seep through the cotton pads. Plus there's the possible danger of them igniting on fire. If you have hot pads like these, consider replacing them with ones lined with asbestos; they are a much safer alternative. That's what the serious home chef should use. Many hot pads, including those with Consumers Union ratings, are available on the market from a number of sources.

If the chef envisions constant peering into an open oven, he or she may also wish to apply a moisturizer or suntan lotion before beginning the oven work.

Eyes

When considering the safety precautions he can take to protect from burns, the home chef should also consider the safety of his eyes, as eye injury can result from a number of incidents in the kitchen. For example, a cork can turn into a dangerous object when projected, at fast speeds, from the bottle of vintage champagne into someone's eye.

Burns of the eyes require the same treatment as a bleeding eye. As discussed previously, lightly cover the eyes with a sterile or clean towel or cloth and immediately dial 9-1-1 and/or head for the emergency room. Examination and treatment by professional ophthalmologist is immediately called for; an eye burn is extremely serious and requires expert attention ASAP.

But fire isn't the only substance to watch out for. Various chemicals, such as those used to unclog drains or garbage disposals or scour tile kitchen counter tops, can also be extremely dangerous if used improperly.

In the case of a burn caused by a chemical agent, water is the immediate first-aid solution. The burnt area should be placed under the tap in the kitchen sink and irrigated with cool running water for at least a quarter of an hour. If the chemical has gotten into the eye or eyes, water should be poured into the eye. Needless to say, once again, in the event of an eye injury, get immediate professional emergency help. Dial 9-1-1 or head immediately to the nearest emergency room or an emergency facility. Many chemical products list emergency care instructions and warnings on their labels. Read the label and see what's recommended as a treatment or antidote.

Lastly, as with heat burns, the burnt area ultimately should be covered with a sterile gauze pad or clean towel or cloth.

It's advisable that the home chef has at the ready somewhere in the kitchen a small fire extinguisher. This could prove useful in the event of total havoc and a raging blaze. While fires can occur in the kitchen from liquids and sauces boiling over onto the hot coils or gas of the range, or by something incinerating in the oven, danger can also lurk elsewhere. For example, a wooden counter top could be set ablaze accidentally as the home chef caramelizes the crusty top of a crème brûlée with a small kitchen blowtorch or ignition of cognac atop a Baked Alaska, plum pudding or crepe suzette, which are not safe activities.

Also, watch those candles. They create a wonderful ambiance for dining but remember, they're fire. We once observed, in a tony mid-Manhattan, Italian restaurant, a basket of large, thin, flat bread go up in flame because the waiter placed the basket, with its overflowing bread leaves, too close to the low-lying candles on the table. The flames shot room high and had to be quickly extinguished with a large bottle of sparkling water.

Thus, too, watch that cigarette smoking in the kitchen. A misplaced smoke or ash amidst various combustibles, gas, inflammable liquids and fats can set the whole place ablaze.

Should the chef himself or herself catch fire—for example, a toque sleeve flares up in smoke—the chef should get down on the floor and roll over on the ignited material, and smother it. Should a guest's or sous chef's kitchen or dining apparel go up in flames, the victim should be placed on the floor and told to roll over and over. Additionally, the chef should smother the flames with a blanket, a thick coat or jacket, or a tablecloth.

Frostbite

Uncommon, but possible given the age of the chef and the use of prescription medications and alcohol, frostbite could occur in the kitchen. That's because if the kitchen is a locus of heat and flame, it's also an environment where exposure to ice and cold is often prevalent. This will be immediately obvious to anyone who has tried to take ice cubes out of the fridge with wet hands. There's a distinct possibility that the ice may stick to the hand, causing cold-related injury. The same holds true for bags of frozen vegetables and the like.

The most extreme cold-inflicted injury in the kitchen could be frostbite. Frostbite occurs when the skin and/or the bodily tissues under the skin freeze. It can occur in just a few minutes. Symptoms of mild frostbite are a blanching or whitening of the skin. Severe cases can appear waxy-like with a white, grayish-yellow or grayish-blue color. Stinging, burning, numbness, firmness and pain are generally present.

As with all other serious injuries, and frostbite certainly qualifies as one, immediate professional medical attention is required. In addition to skin injury, there's also a danger of infection, so a chef or guest with frostbite needs immediate medical examination.

As first-line treatment in the home, the injured area should start to be rewarmed. An appropriate warming technique, according to medical authorities, is to use a tub of water at 100° F (38-40° Celsius) for 30 to 45 minutes (warm to the touch but not hot) until the area gets a good red flush to it. This can be painful, as the skin goes through stages of thawing. If a tub isn't available, warm wet packs at the same temperature can be used.

Don't use dry heat, such as a sunlamp, radiator or heating pad, to thaw the affected area. And don't massage the injured area; it may cause more injury. Once thawed, the injured part should be kept on a sterile gauze or sheet and elevated. Analgesics such as non-steroidal anti-inflammatories may be administered for pain. Frostbitten victims should neither use alcohol, nicotine nor other drugs that may affect blood flow.

Precautions and preventive measures

- Remember: think before you act.
- Always use pot holders.
- Make sure your hands are dry when taking ice or other very cold items from the refrigerator or freezer. Use gloves, if necessary.
- Throw out any food that comes in contact with broken glass.
- Slice away from you, never toward you.
- Never have the knife-edge or blade pointed toward you, always away. Never poke anything you're holding in your hand with a sharp pointed utensil. If you're going to poke or impale anything, put it on the kitchen counter or a cutting board or plate. The same for slicing, such as when slicing cheese.
- Always make sure your fingers are sufficiently away from the part or section that's being cut. Take your time, don't rush.
- Always use properly sized knives and utensils, and use them in the right manner. For example, do not use a large cleaver to whack off potato slices.

- Handle fish bones and spiny vegetables—such as the artichoke—with respect and care.
- Always stack knives and forks downside in the dishwasher, utensil drainer or sink drainer.
- Throw out any food that may have become contaminated with glass.

III

Broken Bones, Muscle Strains and Spine Injuries

The evening promises to be grand. You've invited to tonight's dinner several of your closest friends. The house is warm and inviting. A Purcell concerto with piano and trumpet stirs the air, as you, glass wine goblet filled with a noble deep, rich red burgundy, go about making a beef roulade. Your synchronized movement amid the set and setting of the kitchen is a spectacle no less worthy than that of a premiere ballet.

Yet, waiting offstage, behind the curtains and props, lurks a sinister fiend, one of many that haunt fine dining establishments the world over, from the smartest home kitchen to the four-star Michelin restaurant. Here, we speak of carpal tunnel syndrome, the bane of secretaries, typists, computer workers and assembly line workers.

Carpal tunnel syndrome is also referred to as repetitive strain injury. It's caused by repeated use of the wrists, and it can be painful, running from numbness and tingling in the fingers to pain in the hand, wrist and forearms. It's caused by the pinching of a nerve in the wrist by muscle ligaments.

Repetitive stress injury to the wrist is more often to occur in the home kitchen when the chef is preparing large portions from scratch that require a lot of handwork. For example, a meal that requires peeling, slicing and dicing twelve large potatoes and chopping two bunches of leeks for a vichyssoise, or a meal that requires slicing and chopping zucchinis, onions, ginger, and chicken for a sizzling stir-fry. Another common cause of carpal tunnel syndrome in the kitchen occurs when scrubbing pots and pans or when scraping off a range top or burner with heavily baked-on food with a knife or steel wool.

There are also longer-term palliatives for chronic repetitive stress syndrome, and a physician should be consulted for recommended treatments. Exercise and rest are the home chef's best bets to cope with this affliction, so as to be able finish off the meal with the same zest and zeal with which the preparation started. Here, however, we address what might be done as a first-line action to cope with the aches and pains of repetitive stress syndrome as they present themselves in the home kitchen during meal preparation.

When confronted with a large amount of chopping and slicing, it's advisable to change the position of your hand from time to time as you peel, slice and mince away. It's also advisable, as in many other kitchen operations, not to rush. Leave plenty of time, and give yourself a break now and then by resting your hands for five to ten minutes. Simply lay your wrists on the kitchen counter top.

Also, place your hands in line with your forearm as you go about your chefferie. In other words, keep your wrists and hands in a straight line with your arms. Do not bend the wrists backward or forward.

For immediate pain relief, a natural remedy most likely exists in your refrigerator. A bag of frozen peas or ice. Wrap the peas in a towel or large washcloth and apply the compress to the injured area for ten minutes. Pain relievers such as ibuprofen, naproxen, aspirin or acetaminophen are also helpful and should be available in the kitchen medical chest. Ibuprofen or naproxen are preferable in that, as anti-inflammatories, they can help loosen strained muscles and reduce swelling, as well as alleviate the associated pain.

Broken bones

Carpal tunnel syndrome is not the only casualty among a multiplicity of spine and muscle strains and bone breaks that can occur in the kitchen. These can range from a sore back or spine due to long hours spent on your feet, to cramped hand and arm muscles due to chopping, mincing, or whisking, to a pulled back muscle from lifting a large pot of roast or turkey into or out of the oven.

In fact, one of the most debilitating accidental occurrences that can occur in the home kitchen is when a chef drops a heavy object—such as a roast pot from the oven, a heavy automatic breadmaker, etc.—and it falls on a foot, thus breaking it. Another not infrequent occurrence could be slipping and falling on something spilled on the floor, with a resultant break of arm, leg or other appendage.

Needless to say, a broken arm, foot or leg requires immediate medical emergency attention. The home chef, guest or other individual in the kitchen should call paramedics (9-1-1) or the victim may be taken immediately to the nearest hospital, emergency room or medical clinic and receive professional attention and care.

In the interim, if at all possible, it's extremely important not to move the broken limb, appendage, or person, unless absolutely necessary. This is especially critical if a head, neck or back injury is involved or suspected. The reason is that broken bones, whether they be internal or exposed through the skin, can lead to a variety of numerous complications. These can range from infection to paralysis to severing or cutting internal nerves, organs or arteries or blood vessels.

Two guiding rules apply to bone breaks or fractures:

The first, get immediate professional medical emergency assistance. Dial 9-1-1 or any other immediate medical emergency response unit and/or head right for the emergency room or emergency medical facility.

The second, if you in any way *think* a bone is broken, act like it is. It is best here to err on the side of conservatism.

As with cuts and punctures, if the bone is protruding through the skin, apply a sterile gauze, clean towel or other clean cloth over the rupture and stop the bleeding.

If the individual is to be moved, the broken bone should be secured with a splint to keep the bone from moving. A simple splint can be made from a piece of wood, tied by wide pieces of cloth. In the event these are not available, placing cardboard from a cardboard box or a wad of newspaper pages around the injured area and securing those with pieces of cloth or even trouser belts can make a temporary splint (Diagram A). Cloth padding, or a blanket or a towel, should be placed within the roll of thick paper or cardboard for comfort and further security. In the event strips of cloth are needed, don't be finicky about ripping up a good towel, napkin or tablecloth.

A sling should also be devised from a large cloth to keep forearms, wrists or hands from moving. The chef can make a sling out of any large cloth, part of a tablecloth, a large towel, or a shirt. The cloth should be folded over into a triangle. The elbow of the arm should be placed in the fold of the triangle and the two loose ends tied together around the victim's neck. The arm should ultimately rest in the folded cloth against the victim's stomach.

Finger and toes can be secured by taking a small piece of wadded or balled cloth, or a cotton ball, and inserting it between the broken finger or toe and an adjoining digit that isn't broken. Roll some adhesive tape over the two, securing them together.

Lower legs can be secured by the use of a rolled blanket in the same manner as the newspaper used for arm breaks. But just like in the case of broken toes or fingers, wrap the blanket around the injured leg and then tie the blanketed leg to the person's good leg. Obviously, the individual will have to be carried to the emergency room. If the chef has a broomstick or broom sticks available, these also could be employed to fashion temporary leg splints.

Breaks involving the upper legs and hips should wait for the paramedics or emergency medical teams to be tended to. These breaks should not be moved. If they must, wooden splints must be fashioned to reach from the armpit to the foot and from the waist or groin to the foot. They must be padded and secured.

A simple, temporary emergency splint from newspaper

Diagram A

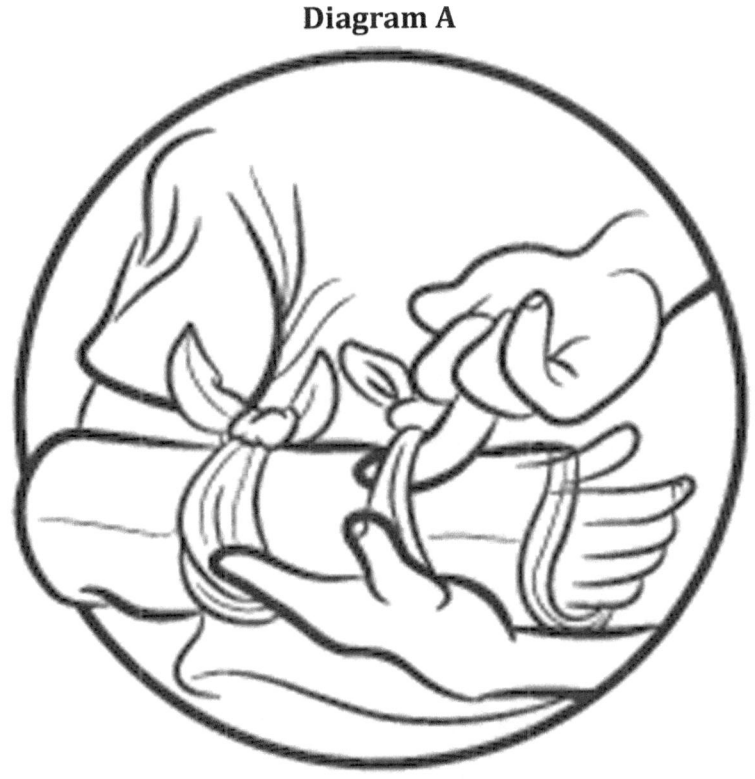

Muscle strains

The home chef who's prepared a chicken for *fricassée*, or beef or lamb or a *pot-au-feu* is already familiar with anatomy because a lot of the anatomy of animals is similar to that of humans. No doubt the home chef has, when, say, preparing chicken, tussled with the gristly muscle adjoining bones. This is a ligament, a tough band of muscle tissue that connects a bone's joint to the muscle that operates it.

Sometimes, when under force or pressure, these ligaments get pulled or stretched too tightly and produce pain, swelling or even bruising. Sprains are particularly common in the wrists, fingers, knees and ankles. Common ways sprains in the home kitchen can occur to the fingers, for example, when opening tight lids on peanut butter, jelly or tomato sauce jars, opening tin cans with a can opener, forcing open jars and bottles, or lifting heavy objects such as roasting pans.

Mild strains can be tended to by placing ice wrapped in a towel or napkin over the injured area. A bag of frozen peas or vegetables can be used instead of the ice. An elastic bandage, available at pharmacies and hospital supply stores, can be used to support the strain. You should start to wrap the bandage below the strained area and work upward. No home kitchen should be without an elastic bandage or two in its emergency medicine chest (Chapter 14).

In any event, severe strains need prompt professional medical attention. A severe strain or sprain can be characterized as any sprain or strain where a sound may be heard, such as "crack," "pop," or "rip." These should be treated as seriously as a broken bone, as a muscle or ligament, for example, may have torn. No need to dally, get to the emergency room.

The back

Most back and muscle injuries occur in the kitchen because of some odd movement the chef makes: an odd turn here, a twist there, a pivot here. Improper lifting techniques can also take their toll (yes, there are proper ways to lift heavy objects). When lifting a pot of roast, a large pan of suckling pig or a plate of whole sea bass, for example, remember to hold your arms steady, bend your knees, and lift the assemblage with your knees. Don't try to yank the heavy pot out of the oven with your torso or your arms by themselves; you'll be asking for trouble.

Much back pain expresses itself in the lower back. Like other medical conditions, lower back pain can, in some instances, be a symptom of a more severe underlying medical cause. Should numbness or weakness occur in the lower back or other limbs, dial 9-1-1 or head for the emergency room, as there may be damage to the nerves involved. Having said that, we are here only here interested with back pain that is directly related to kitchen activity where the action and the body's reaction are clearly identified.

Severe back pain, from lifting heavy pots or just standing on one's feet for hours while making a meal, can be reduced by applying an ice pack to the affected area—as aforementioned, ice wrapped in a plastic bag or a towel may be used, instead. It will also help reduce any swelling in the muscle. Also, pre-made ice packs are available in drugstore and pharmacies. They can be kept in the refrigerator and used over an over again. An ice pack should generally be applied for about a quarter of an hour, every hour.

As with other muscle pains, ibuprofen, naproxen, aspirin or acetaminophen are all good pain relievers. Ibuprofen and naproxen are particularly recommended, since they are non-steroidal anti-inflammatories, and will help relax the muscle, as well as reduce or alleviate pain.

If your back is really aching, a good method to ease pressure is to lie down flat out on the floor on your back. Raise your knees and prop your lower legs with pillows or a rolled up blanket.

Sometimes, during extended heavy-duty work on your feet, back pain can combine with carpal tunnel syndrome, an agonizing combination. Here, too, a rest on the floor, with hands relaxed at your sides, can offer relief.

Good posture is also important to help ease back strain. The home chef, for his gastronomical workout, may wish to procure a simple elastic back brace, available in pharmacies and drug stores, to wrap around his waist if long periods on the feet are required for meal preparation. In severe cases, heavy-duty braces, the kind worn by furniture movers, might be suggested. These are readily available for purchase.

Proper shoes are also critical to good posture and less wear and tear on the feet, ankle and leg muscles. Shoes with non-slip bottoms and good insoles are recommended. Sneakers are a good choice. Thick floor mats of rubber or sponge, used for industrial, commercial, and certain sports, such as weightlifting, are also available. They ease lower back and leg stress and fatigue, and help provide better blood circulation.

Lastly, for the sake of your back and other limbs, make sure your kitchen has a non-slip floor surface. If it doesn't, you can wax the floor with a non-slip wax. At any rate, be sure not to wax your kitchen floor with a wax with a slippery finish.

Preventive measures

- Use a rubber opener to open tight lids on bottles and jars.
- When lifting a pot of roast, a large pan of suckling pig or plate of whole sea bass, remember to hold your arms steady, bend your knees, and lift the assemblage with your knees. Don't try to yank the heavy pot out of the oven with your torso or your arms by themselves.
- Wear comfortable shoes with non-slip bottoms and good insoles, or sneakers.

IV

Choking and Asphyxiation

Choking and asphyxiation are serious medical emergencies that can easily happen to the chef in the kitchen or the guest in the dining room. It's the one dangerous activity in the dining room that is most closely associated with eating: stuffing too much food into one's mouth. And the better and tastier the cuisine, the greater the probability of occurrence.

Anyone practicing the art of home cuisine should be familiar with what to do when, for example, a very common occurrence in restaurants, an inebriated or enthusiastic diner ingests too large a piece of food into his or her mouth and swallows.

While choking and asphyxiation can be caused by many different medical conditions—and there could be numerous underlying causes involved—we are addressing only the immediate emergency diagnosis of an obstacle, typically a food substance, be it a ball of masticated meat or pasta, in the airway passage. The immediate objective is to unblock the airways by removing the obstacle to obtain unobstructed breathing.

In the event of choking or asphyxiation, time is of the essence. Medical literature shows that a person can go without breathing for but one to two minutes. Signs of asphyxiation include blueness of face, rapid pulse, heavy sweats, and bulging eyes.

Some restaurants, because of the commonality of this emergency and the necessity to take immediate action, post signs of the Heimlich maneuver on the walls of their restaurants or in the kitchens.

The Heimlich maneuver was named after Dr. Harry J. Heimlich, a U.S. thoracic surgeon. The steps are completed as follows: first, grab the victim from behind in a bear hug with one of your hands made into a fist. Make sure the thumb side of the fist is placed in the middle of the stomach, above the navel and below the ribs. Then take the fist in your other hand and grasp it tightly. Forcefully and quickly, pull upward into the stomach five times—like jerking upward. If the food doesn't come out, try again.

The Heimlich Maneuver

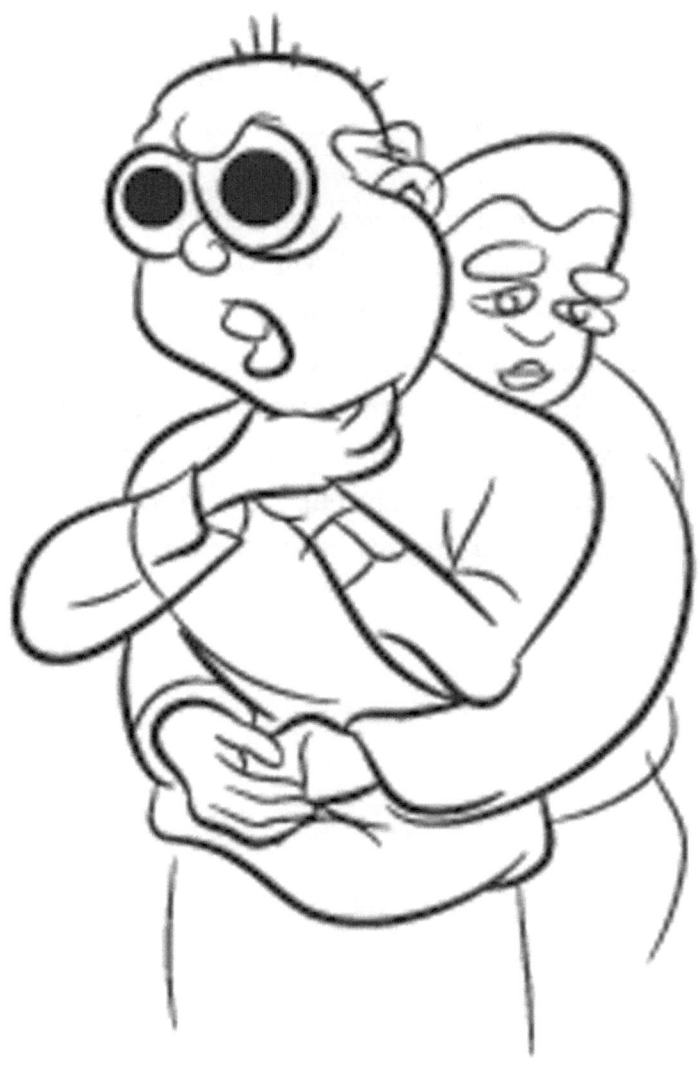

You may wish to tear the full-page diagram of the Heimlich maneuver (previous page) from this book and post it on the side of your refrigerator or similar place.

The key thing to be aware of in a choking incident is whether the person is getting enough air. It's possible to see if the person is breathing, as when the person is able to cough or talk. If the person can't get any air, use the Heimlich. As a first step, prior to performing a Heimlich, the individual should be encouraged to cough to see if the food wad can be coughed up. Choking, which cuts off the supply of oxygen, can quickly lead to asphyxiation. Signs of asphyxiation include bulging eyes and a bluish face, high-pitched wheezing and an inability to cough or speak or breathe.

At worse, the person can sink into unconsciousness.

In the event of any of these serious conditions, 9-1-1 must be called immediately, and/or emergency medical advice must be sought immediately from the emergency room, doctor or paramedic. Time is of the essence.

Should the person lose consciousness while the chef or a helper is calling 9-1-1, the person should be placed face up in the floor or another hard, supportable surface. As a first step, look in the mouth and see if there's anything there that can be removed by your fingers. (See stuck bones on page 34.) Step two: tilt the head back and lift the chin up to open the airway.

If the person is not breathing, try to resuscitate him or her with your own breathing, by forcing air into the person's lungs. With one hand, pinch the person's nose shut. Seal your mouth over the person's mouth. Breathe long and hard into the person's mouth. This should be long and hard enough so that you can see the person's chest rise. If this doesn't work, tilt the person's head back more and try again a couple of times.

If that doesn't work, try a supine Heimlich: straddle the person with your legs, putting the heel of your hands in the middle of the stomach just below the ribs and above the navel. Put your other hand on top of the hand on the stomach and quickly and forcefully thrust upward into the stomach toward the person's head. Try this five times.

Failing this, and if you do not see the chest rising, check the mouth again, and the do five thrusts and two breaths into the mouth. Keep doing this until professional medical help arrives, such as a paramedic team or ambulance.

For this reason, comfortable familiarity with the Heimlich is necessary and, for the chef who cooks and entertains a lot, dry runs and practice drills, say, with a family member, could be an easy way to become familiar with this useful tool in the event of a tension-filled moment of a medical emergency. It's recommended that any serious home chef who does a fair amount of entertaining have handy in the kitchen a card showing how to perform the Heimlich, as well as a cardiopulmonary resuscitation diagram (Chapters 4 & 11, respectively) for easy and immediate reference.

Stuck bones

Another most common source of choking and asphyxiation in the home kitchen or restaurant is the lodgment of a bone in the throat or windpipe. This can range from a sharp fish bone impaled into the roof of the mouth cavity, to a larger fish bone or chicken bone lodged in the windpipe itself.

While the Heimlich could be attempted in this situation, it may not work because the bone or object may be stuck (like a fishbone, for example) into the epidermal layer of the throat. Thus, it must be extracted.

For emergencies of this type, every home kitchen should be equipped with a pair of surgical pliers and tongs. These are thin, long-nosed, stainless steel surgical forceps used in hospitals and doctors offices and medical clinics. They can be obtained at any medical supply store. It is also imperative that the kitchen emergency cabinet be equipped with a flashlight—preferably a slim, high-intensity, long-stemmed flashlight that you might have seen your doctor use when examining your throat or eyes. This is necessary in order to peer into the throat for precise guidance of the forceps. A tongue depressor is also a useful tool to have on hard in this instance. Inexpensive medical flashlights and tongue depressors are also available from medical supply stores.

In a pinch, should a forceps not be handy, longneck or gooseneck pliers from the garage can be used to extract the object. Remember, though, to sterilize, in alcohol or suitable antiseptic, gritty or dirty pliers from the garage before inserting in the mouth to prevent later complications of infection and disease.

Home alone

Ahhh! You've been working all afternoon in the kitchen on a deconstructed couscous. The chicken is basted to a tantalizing ochre gleam. The wine, a 1992 Grgich Chardonnay, is going to be a superb complement to this nouvelle—no, not nouvelle, but actually postmodernly-prepared North African dish. You know because you've been sampling a bottle as you work—to bring out the inspiration that beats in the heart of the great chef you know you are. Why, to assure authenticity of the meal, you've even made your own pita bread.

Thinking of the pita—it's a while yet before dinner, at least an hour and a half before the guests arrive—you feel your stomach growl. Hunger has built up over the hours at the counter top, and as you check the seasoned rice for the tenth time, you grab a piece of the warm pita from the oven and thrust a large hunk it into your mouth. Suddenly, you begin to choke and wheeze, tears streaming from your eyes. You gasp for air.

The wife is still at work. The children are at school. And you're having trouble breathing. What to do?

As with all medical emergencies in the kitchen, dial 9-1-1 or a medical emergency unit or facility as a first act, providing you can, even if you can't speak.

Then, as a next immediate step, go to a mirror. Open your mouth and look in. If you can see what's stuck, pull it out. If you can't see it, don't try to maneuver your fingers way down your throat, because if you ultimately can't grab it, it may drop farther down.

Failing results, you must perform a Heimlich maneuver on yourself.

As with performing the Heimlich on another person, make a fist with one hand and put it into the middle of your stomach. It should go between the ribs and the navel. Take your other hand and put it over the fisted hand. Then, using the unfisted hand thrust forcibly and quickly the fisted hand up and into your stomach. The object, in this case, a wad of pita, should pop out.

Another method of administering a self-Heimlich is to use the back of a chair or some other hard, firm support. Stand behind the chair, placing the top back of the chair against your stomach, halfway between the ribs and the navel. The height can be adjusted by tilting the chair. Bend over the chair back, and press your stomach against it forcibly. Here, again, the wad, chunk, or object should pop out. (See diagram on page 38).

While not exhaustive, here are the main types asphyxiation that can potentially occur in the kitchen accidentally and what to do about them.

The Self-Heimlich Maneuver

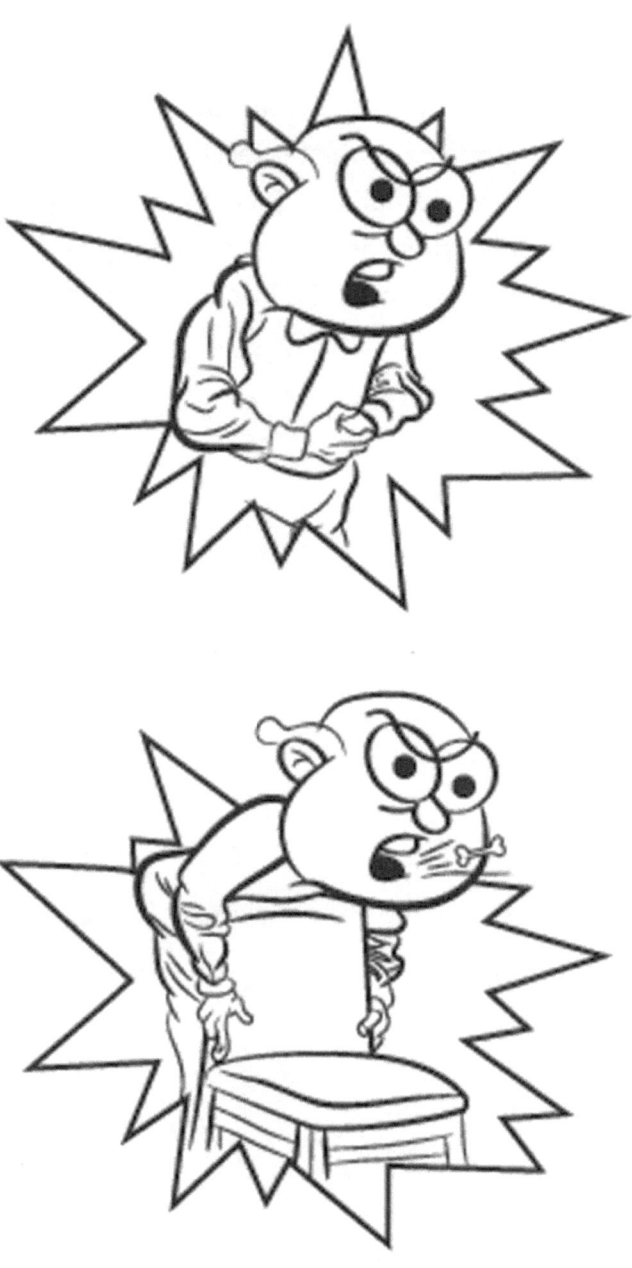

Strangulation

As a general rule, any rotating device in the kitchen presents a potential, and possible, life-threatening hazard. These include garbage disposals, electric mixers, automatic bread makers, electric juicers, coffee bean grinders, and electric can openers.

For this reason, a rule of thumb for the home chef is not to have any loose pieces of clothing dangling from his or her personage. While it may sound bizarre, an all too common medical emergency in the kitchen is when a necktie gets caught in a whirling garbage disposal as the home chef is leaning over the sink. The action is so rapid that the head and neck are drawn down to the sink level so fast that there's no time to deactivate the disposal switch, which is usually on a wall a short distance from the sink. This type of accident, as is the case with just about all accidents, occurs when the chef is distracted under the pressures of time or performing multiple tasks among plates, pots, cooking and steaming and so forth. Most often this is the case when the chef has returned home from a full day of work at the office and is hurriedly duplicating the latest recipe that he or she perhaps saw the Naked Chef make the other night on the cooking channel. Too many distractions: the sure setting for carelessness and danger.

While there's little chance that any body part will enter the disposal, the immediate action is to stop its operation by turning off the switch. However, this alone, will not necessarily insure survival from asphyxiation or other serious damage caused by lack of oxygen.

In the event of this type of emergency, the IMMEDIATE action is to, with a knife or scissors, cut the tie away from the person.

This can be anywhere where a sharp knife blade or scissors can be inserted: at the juncture of the disposal well and the neck, or at the rear of side of the collar.

From a preventive standpoint, it is recommended that the serious home chef always wear a kitchen apron while cooking and cleaning up in the kitchen. Or, if one prefers, a toque of the type professional restaurant chefs wear. It's not so they look like chefs, but because of the protection they afford from heat, splatters, spills and so on. Needless to say, all loose clothing, such as hanging neckties, open, dangling sleeves, collars, scarves and hanging necklaces or bracelets, should be removed before entering the kitchen. A number of smart and attractive kitchen aprons and toques are available for home use and can be purchased directly from a store, by mail or the Internet.

Preventive measures

- Either don't eat or be observant of how you are eating if you are drunk, inebriated or have had a lot of alcohol. Choking on a juicy, man-sized chunk of T-bone or New York strip steak is a classic that all restaurateurs are familiar with.
- Don't talk or laugh with your mouth stuffed full of food.
- Make sure you cut your food, particularly hard or firm items, into small or smallish pieces.
- Be sure to adequately chew the food in your mouth. If you need to make it softer, masticate it with a small sip of water, wine or other beverage.
- Take your time. Eating is to be enjoyed. Right? Savor your meal, the texture, the spices or herbs, the seasonings, the

aroma. Don't eat rapidly, and certainly don't bolt or wolf down big chunks of food. It's bad for your digestion, it ruins the fine dining experience, and you may choke.

- Refrain from wearing loose or dangling clothing while cooking in the kitchen. It's advisable you remove neckties, scarves and dangling jewelry.
- Always wear an apron or toque when preparing large meals.
- Practice the movements of the Heimlich maneuver with a family member or friend, to get the feel of it.

V

Allergic Reactions

Not too long ago, we had the pleasure of hosting a dinner in honor of our 25th wedding anniversary. A special occasion, we took out the fine linen lace tablecloth, the sterling silver dinnerware and porcelain plates. The main course, selected from the *Larousse Gastronomique* and reprinted in the Fall edition of *Bon Appetite* magazine, was a lamb ragout, lovingly braised in the pot, identical to the same peasant dish we had sampled in Provence on a wonderful vacation two years ago to the south of France.

We had invited twelve of our dearest and closest friends for a night of bonhomie and romantic nostalgia. The wine selected from our modest but carefully selected cellar was a 1975 Chateau Lafite Rothschild Grand Cru cabernet sauvignon.

A warm fire ablaze in the hearth, we gathered in good and hearty cheer at the dinner table as the wine was poured and several toasts were given. As the last toast was uttered, and a warm blush crossed our cheeks, Arthur A., who was sitting toward the end of the table, began to cough violently and gasp for air. Water and pats on the back were offered to no avail, as Arthur's coughing became louder and louder and spasmodic. Quite a turn of events on what was supposed to be the loveliest dinner of our lives!

As we were to discover, with Arthur resting comfortably in an upstairs bedroom, the dregs of the wine bottle had been poured on the last toast, the very last drops tenderly poured into Arthur's wide crystal goblet. Unbeknownst to any of us at the table, the dregs of the bottle contained, from years of sitting on the shelf awaiting this special moment, a concentration of sulfites—a naturally occurring chemical that Arthur A. was allergic to.

This incident, fortunately resolved in Arthur's favor, illustrates a type of common medical emergency that occurs more often these days in home kitchens and restaurants than in previous times. In times gone by (actually not that long ago), basic foodstuffs were obtained in the region where people lived. In other words, foods more or less indigenous to the area. Today, our food can come from anywhere, and we emphasize anywhere, in the world on short notice. Foodstuffs, raw, fresh, prepared or preserved, travel overnight by air. Moreover, in the American economy, as many other advanced countries, there is a greater abundance and variety of food and foodstuffs available to the population than at any other time in man's history. Not only in restaurants, but the produce and foods we buy daily in the supermarket or grocery store, as a visit your local produce section will amply demonstrate. Tangerines from Brazil, escarole from Ecuador, tomatoes from Mexico, lotus roots from Indonesia, nuts from Thailand. There are over 200 types of single-malt scotch alone. And who knows how many microbrews from specialty beer microbreweries?

On the one hand, people, because they haven't grown up with the foods as part of their local or natural diet, my not be able to handle them allergically. Also, the combination of strange, different and exotic plants and vegetables may produce unusual and unexpected allergic reactions.

An allergy is a response of the body's immune system to a molecular foreign invader, a pathogen. We're most familiar with a sneeze, which is the body's way of ridding the invader from the nose, and ultimately system.

As we have seen, not all immune reactions or allergies can stem from microbes or viruses, as one might commonly think. They can be triggered by a number of foreign elements, organic or inorganic: chemicals, fabrics, sunlight, and many more. And depending upon what the offending element is, the body's immune system can attempt to combat it in a variety of ways, thus symptoms begin to appear. Sometimes symptoms can manifest themselves in the skin, as is the case with hives, or sneezing, burning eyes, burning sensations, exotic manifestations like *pueritis annitis* (induced by chocolate), or as in Arthur A.'s case, coughing and muscle constriction.

Like a restaurateur or food manufacturer, or perhaps even more so, the home chef entertaining guests has a special responsibility to be aware of what his guests are dining on. It is only in recent years that allergic reactions to peanuts were discovered to be widespread. This has resulted in the decision of many food companies to be more strict on labeling products containing peanuts, restaurants noting food ingredients on their menus, and even airline companies banning free peanuts on airplanes. So if the home chef is going to prepare a masterpiece with organic leche nuts from the Amazon, he or she should learn from this example and politely alert their guests.

From a scientific and purely medical standpoint, the modern kitchen is a witch's den full of strange chemicals, artificial seasonings and odd and unusual foodstuffs that can cause a multiplicity of allergic reactions. It would do well for the serious chef to be familiar with at least some of these and how to deal with them. Allergies, as we've noted, can stem from a number of sources and causes. Here, we deal only with those that might be kitchen and cuisine-related.

Eggs, milk, nuts and seafood are most common food allergic reactions, although probably most anything can cause an allergic reaction based on a person's genetic makeup, for example, the odd case in which a sesame seed mixed into a plain roll becomes lethal.

Peanuts, which we've already noted as a major food allergy, and seafood, particularly shellfish, are the most commonly known food allergenics that can bring on immediate, strong, violent and even lethal reactions. Shellfish, in particular, would include shrimp (as in Shrimp Diablo or Divine, or Garlic Shrimp), oysters (as in Oysters Rockefeller), mussels (as in green New Zealand mussels), crab (New England crab cakes), or lobster (Lobster Bisque Soup). Obviously, anyone with a known seafood allergy should be wary of sushi or sashimi plates.

The most serious allergic reaction results in oxygen being cut off as the throat swells shut and closes. This is called anaphylactic shock. Anaphylactic shock can be brought on by a variety of substances, such as bee stings, but here we are only concentrating on matters related to food and the kitchen.

Allergic food shock shows the same symptoms as other types of shock: hot reddened skin on the face or elsewhere, intense itching or hives or bumps, rapid swelling of the tongue or face, wheezing and troubled breathing, rapid heartbeat, dizziness, stomach cramps, nausea, vomiting, or even passing out.

In the event of severe allergic reaction or anaphylactic shock, call 9-1-1 immediately and ask for professional medical emergency help or advice. Then, immediately get the person to an emergency medical room or facility.

The most immediate remedy for severe anaphylactic shock is to give the person an antihistamine or a hypodermically administered shot of epinephrine. Since these are not commonly found or necessarily available in many households, the prepared chef should keep an antihistamine or single-dose injectable hypodermic in his or her kitchen medical supply kit (Chapter 14).

In the event a person loses consciousness, every attempt must be made to keep oxygen flowing to the lungs. That means the airway must be kept open. Lay the person on the floor and kneel beside him or her. The person's arm closest to you should be kept straight and tucked under the body. The person's other arm should be placed across his or her chest. The ankle farthest way from you should be placed over the one nearest you. With the person's head in your hand, pull the person over onto his or her side. You can do this with the aid of the person's clothes. As the body rolls, support the body with your knees, so it doesn't just flop over.

Tilt the person's chin backward to open the airway. To prop the body, bend the top arm and knee. This should also help making breathing easier. The bottom arm should be lying straight behind the body, out from under it.

Check to see that the person's breathing. If there's no breath or pulse, you must begin cardiopulmonary resuscitation. See Chapter 11 for a description and diagram of how to perform cardiopulmonary resuscitation, or CPR. It is suggested that this diagram be removed from this book and placed somewhere in the kitchen immediately available, the same as for the Heimlich maneuver.

VI

Dermatological Problems and Skin Care

The home kitchen contains many potential skin hazards. Warm water, heat, soaps, detergents and cooking ingredients all take their toll on the epidermis. All are capable of inducing irritating rashes and itches as well as dry, flaky skin. There are therefore a multiplicity of dermatological problems associated with the kitchen, ranging from the chapped hands that result from washing the dishes to a full-blown eruption of patches of red skin and maddening itching from working with fowl or certain other vegetables.

Most rashes and itches normally clear up on their own. Doctors (dermatologists) have a name for this type of rash or itch: contact dermatitis, which results from coming in contact with something that irritates the skin. This can range from, as we've said, food and soaps, detergents and even other chemicals (such as cleaning solutions) and materials. Generally, red rashes, bumps and blisters distinguish contact dermatitis. They can appear anywhere on the body.

Rashes and itching (including severe dermatitis with oozing pus, scales, craters, and so on) can also result from underlying medical conditions, including stress. Here we are only discussing those rashes and itches that occur immediately in the kitchen upon contract with an irritating or alien substance.

What to do?

Applying hydrocortisone or diphenhydramine can quickly alleviate most rashes and itches that occur from contact in the kitchen. These are antihistamines, which block the production of histamine, which the body produces to combat the irritation, thus producing a rash or itch. Antihistamines are available over-the-counter at your drugstore or supermarket remedy section. We advise that the home chef have a small tube in his kitchen medical emergency kit for him or herself or for any guests who may erupt with an itch or rash.

Try, as you might, do not scratch the offending patch of skin. You don't want to break the skin by scratching because it could make the condition worse. Also, it could lead to infection.

In the event of a skin irritation caused by a chemical of some sort, the chef should first clean the area with soap. Then he or she should place his or her hand under the tap in the kitchen sink and let water run over it for several minutes. Treatment of a contact dermatitis from a chemical should not be confused with a chemical burn or allergic reaction. They are different and should be treated differently than contact dermatitis.

Since most contact dermatitis in the kitchen usually centers on washing dishes, it's advisable that the home chef secure a pair of gloves to use when washing dishes. Thin latex or rubber gloves are readily available in supermarkets, and these are superb for handling chemicals such as those used to scour kitchen counter tops, kitchen tile, or linoleum floors in kitchens. However, they may not be the ticket for all chefs when it comes to using them continually for dishwashing. That's because some people have allergic reactions to latex, a known allergen. Chefs with latex or rubber allergies should seek out gloves that are latex or rubber on the outside, but lined inside with some other material, such as cloth.

For the chef who entertains a lot, to reduce punishment of the hands in the kitchen, he or she should obtain a good moisturizing lotion and apply it at night, or in the morning. This will help keep the wear and tear down on the skin, and help reduce that dried out, wrinkled, white scaly or chapped look to the hands after the meal is over, the guests gone, and the dishes washed.

If the kitchen is exceptionally hot, the chef may wish to invest in a small room humidifier to keep the air in the kitchen moist. This will reduce dehydration and chapping of the face, a sure occurrence if the chef's face goes in and out of the oven checking on baking, grilling or braising. It will also help reduce split or dried out hair caused by blistering heat.

Fingernails can also take a beating when making a meal or cleaning up afterward. Dulled, chipped, and scrapped nails from kitchen work are not serious medical problems. But they certainly present a cosmetic problem. The use of kitchen gloves will help reduce the exposure of fingernails to the hostile climate of the kitchen.

Preventive measures

- Use gloves when washing dishes or scouring the countertop with chemical cleaning solutions.

- Consider using organic or hypoallergenic cleaning solutions for dishwashing.
- Use a good moisturizer on your hands the night before or the morning of the day you are cooking.
- Consider buying a humidifier for the kitchen if the air is always warm and dry.

VII

Infectious Diseases and Food Poisoning

Food poisoning comes from spoiled or rotten food, such as fresh fruits that have been contaminated with bacteria, pesticides or agricultural chemicals.

Most bacteria, viruses and pathogenic organisms harmful to the human body can take between 12 to 48 hours to germinate and erupt into symptoms—long after your luncheon, brunch or dinner party has ended.

We think we live in a safe and sterile world, especially in the United States. But in fact, our food supply is heavily contaminated with chemicals, pesticides, hormones and bacteria of all variety, shapes, sizes and nastiness. According to the literature reports of Physicians Committee for Responsible Medicine, the yearly incidence of foodborne illness range from 6.5 to 81 million people infected. The vast majority of cases they report go undetected. From 1973 to 1987, 7,458 outbreaks, involving 237,545 cases of food poisoning were reported to the Centers for Disease Control and Prevention (CDC). Bacterial infections caused 66 percent of the outbreaks, 87 percent of the cases, and 90 percent of the fatalities. Beef, dairy products, pork and poultry are usually associated with these cases. It's been estimated that some 90 percent of the chickens in the U.S. carry chlamybacter. In 1998, an estimated 8 million cases of foodborne illness occurred, according to the CDC.

According to the CDC, over 200 diseases can be spread through food. The journal of *Emerging Infectious Diseases* (September 1999) reports that some 79 million food-borne illnesses occur in the United States annually. These result in an estimated 325,000 hospitalizations and 5,000 deaths.

This is an extraordinarily good reason to follow the cautions and instructions on every pack of uncooked chicken, eggs, beef and other poultry. Cross-contamination—contamination by contact with infected meat or contaminated utensils or kitchen surfaces—is a persistent danger. Make sure to wipe down, with a sterile solution, cutting blocks, utensils or anything else that may have come in contact with raw, uncooked chicken or raw meats. Any spoiled or cracked chicken eggs should be discarded. Needless to say, all foods should be properly cooked and not undercooked.

In addition, to prevent cross contamination, foods should be kept separate in shopping bags. For example, meats and poultry should be kept separated in bags from vegetables and leafy greens. The same at home in the fridge.

Cases of foodborne infection and food poisoning, if at all suspected, must be treated by the medical profession and immediate professional medical care sought. In addition to a wide variety of serious symptoms and further complications, administration of antibiotics and other prescription pharmaceuticals may be needed.

It's also important to know that there a great many and variety of medical problems that exhibit symptoms of food poisoning, such as nausea, diarrhea and vomiting, as part of the symptomatology. We are here, again, only concerned with the very basics of those that may involve food that can or need to be dealt with during the course of a meal at home. Such conditions as internal parasites, gastric ulcers, cardiovascular or heart disease, all of which may involve nausea, as well as diseases with later-manifesting symptoms, lay outside the realm of this book and are best left, diagnosed and treated by the medical profession.

We, therefore, while cautioning the home chef to observe all proper sanitary rules for food handling around the kitchen and cooking, we concern ourselves here with those food-related pathogens that manifests symptoms in the course of several hours, the length of an average home dinner.

Light cases of food poisoning—from bacteria, viruses or chemicals—can last less than a couple of hours or so. They can erupt during a meal and, if not from the meal itself, coincidentally from or in combination with hors d'oeuvres or something ingested before arrival. Even though it may be of relatively short duration, its effects on the body can be a multi-round blast of diarrhea, vomiting, stomach cramps, and pain, fever chills or dizziness.

Diarrhea

Diarrhea, uncontrollable watery stool, is an unpleasant offshoot of eating that happens when there is an imbalance of water in the intestines. Most diarrhea is self-limiting and unhazardous—expect possibly to clothing—and generally goes away with time. If you find yourself enduring this problem, the best advice is not to take anti-diarrheals, of which there are many available in drugstores and supermarkets, at the initial onset. The body itself, over a relatively short period of time, will rid the system of whatever bacteria or pathogens may be lurking within. Obviously, if it does not go away and presents a lengthy or chronic problem, consult a physician as soon as possible. But for common diarrhea make sure you drink plenty of water or fluids to replace that which is lost in the bathroom to make sure you don't get dehydrated, which can be a whole other severe problem unto itself.

But if you do wish to take an anti-diarrheal, a number are available over-the-counter. They differ in their approaches to the problem, ranging from bismuth sulfate, which attacks the bacteria responsible, to over-the-counter medication which mechanically slows the movement of the intestines. You may also be interested to know that bismuth sulfate, taken beforehand, helps prevent diarrhea.

Botulism

While it's not possible to go into a complete etiology of bacteria, viruses and microbes in this book, one distinct and possible infection—although rare—needs to be flagged. This is botulism, a bacterium. Severe botulism can be fatal and requires immediate attention.

Nausea, vomiting, diarrhea, droopy eyelids, blurry vision, trouble swallowing because of a dry mouth, difficulty breathing and muscle weakness and paralysis characterize botulism infection.

In the event you discern any of these symptoms, it's an immediate and automatic call to 9-1-1 or a medical emergency rescue unit or make an immediate trip to the emergency room of a hospital or medical facility.

Severe chemical poisoning

The same is true of chemical poisoning, whether it be from something that came from the food, or something that was accidentally confused or mixed in with the food.

The symptoms, like botulism poisoning, are not pleasant: vomiting and diarrhea, stomach pain, dizziness, confusion, watery eyes, drooling, sweating and blurred vision.

This, too, requires an immediate and automatic call to 9-1-1, a medical emergency or a poison control center. If you have any idea of what the chemical may be, assuming that it's from the kitchen and not the food itself, look on the label of the product. Quite often, manufacturers will give an antidote for accidental poising or ingestion. You might want to call the manufacturer on a consumer hot line if one is listed. Nevertheless, dial 9-1-1 and/ or get to the emergency room or an emergency medical facility immediately.

Vomiting

Vomiting, the uncontrollable expulsion of food or beverage from the stomach, is another one of those nuisance, and sometimes unavoidable, correlates with eating. Man throughout the ages has known vomiting—from the great gluttonous feasts and bacchanals of ancient Rome to the office drunk who goes overboard at the office Christmas party. Projectile vomiting, on the other hand, is when the vomit, a mixture of food, drink, and stomach and gastric acids and fluids, shoot out like a fire hose. It is an unpleasant experience, both for the victim and anyone standing in close range.

Generally, simple vomiting occurs when the body, the stomach, tells you that you have done something bad. You've drunk too much, eaten too much or eaten something you shouldn't have. A very good example we once observed was a gourmet who sampled a bowl of lamb soup in an ethnic restaurant, something he'd never had before, after rounds of vodka toasting. His body said it had to go. And so it did, in a forceful pressured stream several yards long, neatly hitting the back of a well-napped neck of an innocent victim.

As with common diarrhea, vomiting is self-limiting. Once the body has gotten rid of the offender, peace usually reigns again.

E. coli infection and prevention

Escheria coli (E. coli) is a common bacterium found in the digestive tracts of animals and humans. It can cause a variety of illnesses, from bloody diarrhea to kidney problems and can sometimes be fatal. Generally, people contract E. coli infection from food, water or other items contaminated with infected feces, as well as through cross contamination. Unless preventive sanitary measures are kept, E. coli can accumulate in dishrags, sponges, and wooden cutting boards or counters where small cracks may prevail. A quick, easy and effective way to sterilize these items is to put them in the microwave wet: a wet sponge takes one minute, a dishrag three and a cutting board ten.

Hand washing is imperative to prevent infection. Hands should always be washed before preparing food, during food handling and preparation, and after using the bathroom or changing babies' diapers. Fresh vegetables should be washed and all food should be cooked long and hot enough to kill any bacteria. Steaks and roasts should be cooked a minimum of 145° F; ground meats at least to 160° F; poultry, 180° F for thigh and 170° F for breast meat. A meat thermometer should be used to check the temperature if there's any question.

Preventive measures

- Wash hands thoroughly before and after handling and preparing food.
- Cook meats, poultry and eggs at proper heated temperatures to eradicate bacteria.
- Wash raw vegetables before cooking.
- Wipe down counters, range, sinks and cutting boards with warm soapy water to eliminate bacteria and cross contamination.
- Wash all kitchen utensils and serving plates and glasses before using.
- Disinfect dishrags, dishcloths, sponges and cutting boards in the microwave oven.
- Throw out all spoiled food.
- Do not let food sit out for a long time in heat before serving to avoid spoilage and contamination.

VIII

Flatulence, Bloating, Belching and Heartburn

There's no occurrence more uncomfortable or embarrassing to host or guests than the build up of gas during a festive dinner or luncheon party.

Let's face it. Shakespeare may have said, "A rose by any other name smells just as sweet." But, a fart is a fart. And an indelicate, lingering one at an elegant social gathering can be rancid and ruin the whole evening. Gas, wherever it may erupt in the body, is as natural as eating itself and is always a potential blight on the smooth serving of haute or fine cuisine. The late astronomer and cosmologist Carl Sagan once wrote that the one sure way alien beings, cruising by in space ship, would be able to tell there was life on Earth would be by the large amount of methane gas in the atmosphere. The methane gas, of course, being emitted by all the animals, including humans, on earth on any given day. The average person farts about a half-dozen times a day. Who's to say about cows and pigs and the like? The home chef, as with any other potential medical problem, must be prepared to deal with this natural curse.

Euphemistically referred to as flatulence by the genteel, gas can quickly build up to bursting proportions in the stomach, intestines or colon. This may occur to the point of uncontrollable expulsion of the gas to deflate the uncomfortable feeling, at the least, or relieve excruciating pressure on the internal organs, at the extreme.

Gas is generated in several ways. Ingesting too much air during eating is one. Simply taking smaller mouthfuls of food, eating slowly and not bolting food, chewing adequately and drinking water or another beverage with your mouthfuls can prevent this. So don't gulp your food. But if you gulp a mouthful of air with that heavenly slab of pork chop, if you are alert enough, you can always expel it through your nose, rather than sucking it into the stomach.

The more serious type of gas build up occurs from rapid fermentation in the stomach. Microorganisms can cause food to rapidly ferment in the stomach. For example, those who are lactose intolerant can experience an immediate and almost debilitating gas inflation, complete with bloat, lower colon pressure and eye-crossing headache, immediately after drinking milk or ingesting milk products.

Lactose intolerance is the inability to digest the principal sugar in milk. Some 30 million Americans are prone to the condition. If the lactase enzyme, the enzyme that digests lactose fails to do its job, bacteria in the gut that generate hydrogen gas metabolize it.

The type of food consumed, such as any dish employing a white sauce, or an egg dish, has a distinct bearing on the always-unpleasant odor and the degree of flatulence. Who, for example, in all candor, cannot at some time or another recall the nauseating, sulfurous smell of egg flatulence?

Once again, prevention is the best cure. The chef who's sensitive to his dining guests' needs may politely note that the special dish that's been prepared contains lactose as an ingredient. The chef may also wish to substitute soymilk in recipes if lactose intolerance is a problem. Supermarkets and specialty food stores are evermore frequently carrying organic and soy products, including soymilks in a variety of flavors and cheeses, among others.

Certain fruits, vegetables, such as cabbage, and grains, particularly high-fiber grains, can produce gas. Beans, of course, are notorious for generating gas, often taking the brunt of vegetable jokes. For this reason, if the chef or chefess feels that he or she must serve beans, such as in a Mexican dish or an Italian halibut over white beans, then try to modify the beans so that they have a less volatile effect when consumed. While not foolproof, the use of dried beans (soaked overnight) is a better bet than beans from a can. Also, a special commercial anti-bean gas product, a digestive aid found in drugstores and supermarkets, can be poured into the bean dish. Guests will be none the wiser and, we're sure, appreciative of your efforts to make them less fart prone.

Sugar and artificial sweeteners are also sure-fire gas producers. If you're concerned about enjoying an unembarrassing, odor-free dinner, try not to make recipes that call for the use of these ingredients. However, this may limit dessert presentations.

Most common gas produced in the human body during mealtime consists of methane gas, a product of natural fermentation, or sulfur. The best course of action in the part of the chef or the guest is to politely excuse himself table and expulse the gas outdoors or in a secluded part of the house or the bathroom with the fan on. This generally results in a temporary relief. The stricken guest or chef should be prepared to dispense a gas absorption remedy, such as activated charcoal or a simethicone-containing gas reduction preparation. Both ingredients have been shown to reduce gas by chemical absorption or breaking up large and uncomfortable gas bubbles in the stomach. A number of antiflatulents are available over-the-counter.

Some herbal remedies have also been known to produce success in diminishing gas pain. These include chamomile, peppermint, anise or fennel tea.

If it's possible to leave the room and go to a secluded spot, lying down on the floor on your back can alleviate severe gas pains. Pull your legs up to your chest. This should make it easier to get the gas out of your system.

In a lurch, the following procedure may be used, but not recommended. Methane gas is ignitable and, like gas coming off an industrial smokestack, can be burnt off. In close quarters, where no other means of outdoor escape or expulsion is available without undue embarrassment, especially in mixed dining company, the guest or chef should head for the nearest coat closet. There, with door closed, the victim should bend over, expel gas, and light a match or cigarette lighter and let it burn off odorously. This is not recommended, however, except in an extreme pinch, since there's a distinct danger of igniting the clothing in the closet on fire. Also, it may be added that a cigarette lighter is best employed in this procedure, as sulfur is a component of matches, and, in this case, with the sulphurous odor coming off the match, the cure may be no better than the disease.

Home alone? The answer is really simple. Let 'er rip!

Belching and burping

Extreme gas build up confined solely to the stomach has a similar cause as flatulence. However, the development of methane gas as a product of ingestion isn't necessarily present.

Gas buildup in the stomach, which is usually highly uncomfortable, is generally the result of too much air in the stomach, or a chemical reaction with the food ingested. This necessitates the need for immediate relief by belching the gas through the mouth or nostrils. The pressure of the gas can often make the gesture almost uncontrollable. The odor of the belch can range from neutral (air) to that which has just been ingested, such as onions or garlic.

In a number of societies, such as in the Orient, belching in a host's face is a distinct sign of appreciation of a good meal, and is expected in some quarters. This is particularly true in a multinational setting, where the host chef and the dinner guests do not share the same common language and must relay on hand and body signals.

On the contrary, belching in the host's or guest's face in Western societies is frowned upon and viewed as a sign of disrespect, as well as an embarrassment.

As with flatulence, the guest or host should seek to remove him or herself from the immediate area and discretely emit the gas. Elsewise, the guest may ask the host chef for some palliative to help restrain the buildup as the course of the meal continues. This is true also of bloating, and heartburn.

Thus, the chef's home medical emergency kit should have, in addition to a good, effective antiflatulent, an effective and quick antacid for bloating and heartburn (available over the counter).

Heartburn

Heartburn is, again, one of those unavoidable offshoots of dining well. Like its cousin gas, it comes along with the show.

Heartburn, or acid indigestion, results from eating acidic, spicy or fatty foods, and from drinking alcohol. It can also result from simply eating or drinking too much. There are other causes of heartburn (or gastroesophageal reflux in medical parlance), but here we are concerned only with those that deal with the ingesting and imbibing of good food and drink at the table.

Heartburn, or acid indigestion, is characterized by a burning sensation behind the breastbone, an acidic vomitous taste in the back of the throat or mouth, and/or upper stomach or chest pain. The noisome, uninvited dinner guest—the belch or burp—is also active here and there. Heartburn should not be confused with a heart attack. Sharp pains in the chest that reach into arms and shoulders characterize a heart attack, among other things. Any signs like this demand a call to 9-1-1 and/or a hasty trip to the emergency room.

Heartburn occurs when acid from the stomach, necessary to digest foods, backs up into the lower throat (or esophagus). A number of antacids are readily available in supermarkets, convenience and grocery stores and drugstores. These offer the quickest route to relief. Most of these antacids that are available over the counter are calcium-based, however there are others that chemically halt secretion of stomach acid. The home chef should have a good antacid in his medicine chest for himself and guests.

There are some natural remedies that can be used for immediate relief. The most time-honored is baking soda or bicarbonate of soda. The recipe is a teaspoon of baking soda in one cup of water. The home chef may also wish to try ginger, ginger tea, ginger root capsules or catnip or fennel tea.

While it would be untoward and uncomplimentary to one's cooking for the chef to offer his guests an antacid *before* dining, the chef, himself, may wish to consider taking an antacid prior to eating if he or she is prone to heartburn, as a preventive measure.

Breath odors

Breath odors are a logical consequence of stomach fermentation by bacteria. There are also the natural aromas of the freshly ingested meal that make their way to the surface air. It's a pity that the highpoints of a good meal—such as garlic from a garlic-rich Mediterranean pasta or seafood dish—can be offensive out of context to another person. Dining, too, as much as a social event as it is, is also a private affair. One may talk about a dish, but one doesn't necessarily want to be bathed in the aroma of it from another person, even one who may have eaten the same thing. Like all other by-products of fermentation, the odors can vary in degree and odor, depending upon the food ingested.

The good chef host should have on hand, at mealtime's end, a breath mint of some type to assist guests in this possible embarrassing condition.

In some instances, the chef, who may be preparing a particularly pungent meal, one sure to induce breath odor, may want to consider adding a breath neutralizer to the cuisine. For example, parsley, available dried or fresh in most supermarkets, is a known deactivator of garlic odor.

Odiferous foods include garlic, hot peppers, salami, anchovies, tuna, onions, leeks, alcohol, pepperoni, Liederkranz, Camembert and blue cheeses, and peanut butter, among others.

Preventive measures

- Take small mouthfuls of food. Don't bolt or gulp food.
- Be sensitive to lactose intolerance among guests.
- Be sensitive to the use of beans, sugar and artificial sweeteners in recipes.
- Avoid highly acidic foods.
- Have breath mints on hand after dinner.

IX

Electric Shock

The contemporary kitchen contains numerous devices that run on electricity. These appliances save so much time and labor that they are a blessing to the home chef and a staple of today's kitchen. In short, we take these appliances for granted.

Yet, they are connected to electricity and in the kitchen, in particular, have the potential for the lethal combination of electricity and water. So, a word is in order about what to do in the event of an electrical medical emergency. If it ever happens, it wouldn't be the first time: a chef accidentally dropping an electric can opener into a basin filled with dishwasher, and attempting to retrieve it without first turning off the electricity (because something needed to be stirred in a pan on the stove).

Should a chef become electrocuted, the first course of action is to shut off the appliance. Pulling the plug from the wall socket or shutting off the electricity in the house, the main current, can do this. Generally, wall switches should not necessarily be relied upon, because they often serve only a special wall outlet or two and it may not be the right one. Also, sometimes they don't work.

An electrocuted chef should not be pulled away from the appliance by another person. The electricity will pass on to the other person, and there will be two problems instead of one. If an attempt is to be made, the rescuer should make sure he or she is standing on some electrically insulated object preferably made of rubber, such as a doormat. A telephone book or other large book could be tried in a pinch.

Always remember that if there's an electrical fire involved, never use water or a liquid to attempt to quench it. Try to smother or suffocate it with a foam fire extinguisher, blanket, coat or jacket.

Also, be wary of burns from electricity. They can be deceptive. They tend to go deep into the skin. What may appear to you to be as a first or second-degree burn may actually be a third or fourth-degree burn. The chef should act accordingly: dial 9-1-1 or take a trip the emergency room.

Preventive measures

- Don't pull away an electrocuted chef from the source of electricity unless you're on an insulated surface.
- Never use water to put out an electrical fire. Suffocate it or use a foam fire extinguisher.

X

Ears

The kitchen can be a noisy place. High decibels from appliances, such as electric mixers, loud chatting or a TV from the next room, loud music that the chef has not personally chosen can all be mentally and physically irritating to the ears. Just as important, loud, irritating noises can be distracting to the home chef, preventing him or her from the exactitude and concentration needed for the preparation of fine, haute cuisine. Think of the racket lawnmowers and leaf blowers make outside the kitchen window on a warm summer afternoon. How's a chef to concentrate?

Like other medical symptoms, ringing in the ears, loss of hearing or pain in the ears can be attributable to any number of underlying disease states. We here are only addressing ear problems that are directly connected to cooking. Ear problems that arise coincidentally in the kitchen during meal preparation demand a call to 9-1-1 or a quick visit to the emergency room or a medical facility, as it could be a symptom of something serious, unrelated to chefferie.

A simple palliative to loud or raucous noise is an earplug. Plugging the ears with antiseptic cotton balls is time-honored. However, little, inexpensive, disposable, foam earplugs are available over the counter and are reasonably effective, depending on the noise level. It wouldn't hurt for the home chef to have a couple of sets in his or her kitchen emergency medical kit.

Preventive measures

- Have sterile cotton balls or earplugs on hand.

XI

Cardiopulmonary Resuscitation (CPR)

Cardiopulmonary resuscitation is for any serious medical emergency where the person has stopped breathing, no pulse or heartbeat can be determined, the person is unconsciousness and the skin has turned blue or paled. For example, a drowning victim.

In the event of these symptoms, dial 9-1-1 immediately and get help from an emergency ambulance or paramedic unit with an electric defibrillator and oxygen supply. Also, determine if anyone, whether in the home or nearby—a neighbor, police, firemen or anyone else—has had formal CPR training.

CPR can help save lives in many emergency situations anywhere. We encourage the home chef, if only as an act of good citizenship, to get formal CPR training.

Failing the above and all else, quick action is necessary. If the heart and lungs are stopped, the brain will be deprived of oxygen and fatality can occur. The brain can't be deprived of oxygen for more than a minute cr two. Precautions are necessary, as many of these situations require extra care. Take, for example, the caution employed when applying pressure to broken ribs in the chest.

Here's what to do:

Check the victim's mouth to ensure there's nothing stuck in it or blocking the throat or airway.

Put the person on the ground where he or she is. The person shouldn't be moved, unless necessary, if spine, neck or head injuries are suspected because of possible neurological damage.

Kneel beside the person midway between the head and chest. Check for breathing by putting your ear next to the mouth. Tilt the person's head back to open the air passage.

If there's no breath, with your fingers, pinch the person's nose shut over the nostrils. Keeping the nose clamped shut, seal your mouth over the person's mouth. Breathe into the person's mouth for one or two seconds, carefully watching the person's chest, to see if it is rising and falling. Don't breathe too hard; if air is forced into the stomach instead of the lungs, choking and vomiting can occur. If this doesn't work, try again, with the person's head tilted farther back.

Next, check for a pulse. The best way to do this is by taking two fingers of each hand and feeling on either side of the neck, just below the jaw, between the front of the throat and the long muscle on the side of the neck.

If a pulse is there, that means the heart is beating. Continue breathing into the person's mouth—one breath every five seconds.

If there's no pulse or heartbeat, chest compression is required. (Precautions are necessary, since, for example, care must be taken in applying pressure to broken ribs in the chest).

Here's what to do:

Again, kneeling beside the person, place your hands on the victim's breastbone. Keep your arms straight, your shoulders above your hands. Take your index finger and middle finger of one hand and place it on the declivity where the ribs meet the breastbone. Put the heel of your hand above this spot, on the middle of the breastbone on the side closer to the person's head. Take your other hand, and put it on top of the hand on the breastbone and interlace the fingers of both hands. Tilt the hands up. The objective is to have only the heel of the bottom hand on the person's chest. With arms locked straight and your shoulders over your hands, push straight down. The breastbone should go down one to two inches. (See diagram on page 75).

Release the pressure, but keep your hands in place. Do the compression 15 times, with short thrusts and a very slight pause between each stroke.

Then switch back and forth between breathing into the mouth and compressing the chest. The sequence is two breaths, 15 chest pushes, two breaths, 15 compressions of the chest. Repeat the sequence four times, then check for a pulse. If there's a pulse, the chest compressions can be stopped but continue the breathing assistance until you are sure that the person can breathe alone.

These activities should be carried out until professional medical or emergency help arrives on the scene.

Home alone

If you are home alone and you need CPR, there's a technique that can be attempted to give you enough time to call 9-1-1. This is not a substitute for CPR by trained emergency personnel, but a last-ditch effort to get help.

If you believe you need CPR, you can try two techniques. Self-administered CPR is similar to self-administered Heimlich; the fist is balled into the upper belly or abdomen and thrust upward as the body rocks back and forth over the chair. Another method is to cough as loud and as hard as you can. Keep doing this until you can get on the phone to 9-1-1. The self-induced coughing paroxysm simulates the chest compressions that should be administered by trained rescue personnel.

CPR Diagram

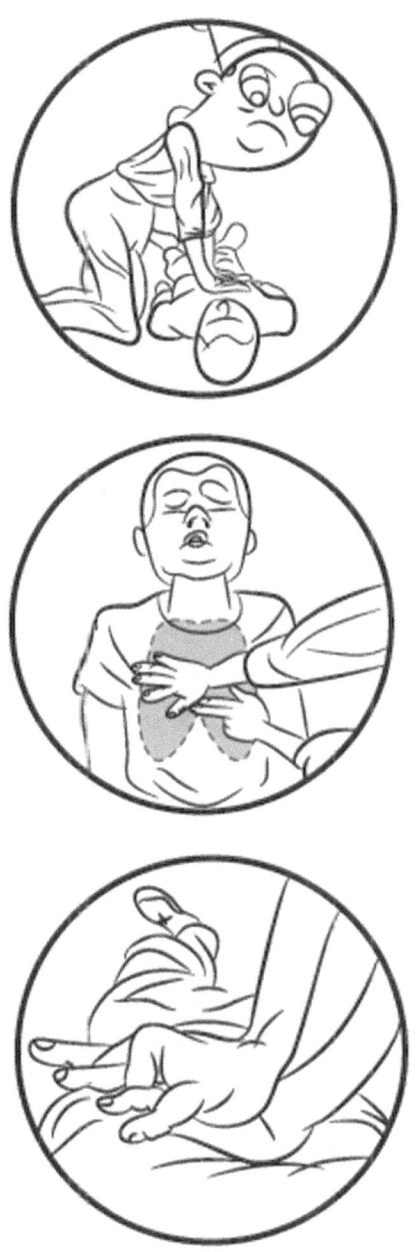

XII

Concussion

Head injuries seem unlikely in the kitchen or dining room, but they can actually happen.

Head injuries can commonly happen when a heavy platter or pot falls from an overhead cabinet or slips from the chef's hands and falls on the chef's head, when the chef slips on a patch of wet floor or a spot where sauce or soup has been spilled. Or even when the chef accidentally slips on wet lettuce leaves from a salad, or portion thereof, that has fallen on the floor. Clunking a head on an open kitchen cabinet door is certainly not unheard of, either.

The dining room, too, can be a danger zone. A laughing or expansive guest, warmed by the delights of the table fare and amicability of the setting, tilts his or her chair backwards and leans back, and clunks his or her head on a sideboard, a china cabinet or the floor. And an intoxicated guest, while making his way unsteadily from the dining table, has been known more than once to lose his balance and fall over and clunk his head on a piece of furniture, say, a glass or marble coffee table.

Head cuts, wounds and bruises should be treated as any other, as described elsewhere in this book.

However, the most important thing to look out for when there's a head injury is the possibility of concussion. Symptoms of concussion, directly linked to getting hit on the head, are dizziness, temporarily loss of consciousness, headache, and nausea or vomiting. If this appears to be the case, the chef should have the 9-1-1 operator on the phone or be on his way to the emergency room or emergency medical facility. Another reason for swift action is that some of these symptoms—dizziness, blurred vision, speech and hearing impairment, confusion—could be a stroke caused by artery damage in the brain.

While waiting for an ambulance, the paramedics or a physician to arrive, the chef (or a guest, if it's the chef who's in trouble) should talk to the victim and try to engage him or her in conversation to alleviate or eliminate what might be a confused state of mind.

It's important not to move the head, neck or spine. There may be neurological damage and further movement could result in paralysis. Put a pillow or rolled blanket or rolled jacket under the head and keep it straight by cradling it in your hands. Loosen the person's clothing and keep him or her warm with a blanket. No food or drink should be given to the victim.

Preventive measures

- Be especially careful removing heavy objects from overhead cabinets.

- Clean up spills of water, liquids and slippery vegetables on the floor right away.
- As with precautions for back injuries, wear shoes with non-slip soles or sneakers.
- Use non-slip wax on the kitchen floor.

XIII

Psychiatric Disorders

Let's face it, part of the allure of home chefism is escape from the daily grind. The home chef seeks the same solace as, say, the weekend gardener by distracting him or herself from the regular routine of work. The aromas, tastes and physical activity of the kitchen offer a rich contrast of experience to the person who sits behind a desk or a computer all day. Because of the availability of a wide range of kitchen equipment and the ready accessibility of exotic victuals, spices, and vinos, the modern kitchen has been a pleasure palace of the senses and, at the extreme, hedonistic—all distractions leading to carelessness and disaster.

In earlier days, the art of imbibing while cooking was politely referred to as "sampling the cooking sherry." Most likely partaken of by Mom or Aunt Millie, whose occasional peculiarities could be attributed to such. However, today, because of the abundance of spirits used in cooking and accompanying gourmet meals, drinking and cooking are right up there with drinking and driving.

The natural dangers that lurk behind imbibing too much alcohol amid fire, flame and sharp objects speak for themselves.

First off, if the chef or anyone is taking drugs, legal or illegal, and sopping up the local vintage in your kitchen, there is a danger signal ahead. We have observed, for example, a food devotee stop in mid-sentence of palaver, stare straight ahead with eyelids completely open and short of breath. While normality returned shortly thereafter, the confession was made that some prescription drug had been involved. In this day and age, chefs, for their own sake, and the sake of their guests, need to constantly remind themselves that alcohol and some foods, such as seasonings and herbs, as well as drugs, do not mix well together.

In fact, if the home chef were to consult a vademacum of natural and homeopathic herbs, he or she would find that many of these herbs contain mind-altering substances. And we're not talking about pot. We're talking about sage, basil, oregano, chamomile or a dozen other herbs that are currently and naturally used in the kitchen, whether it be in restaurants or home kitchens. We're not suggesting that the home chef stop using seasonings, only that he or she be aware of the fact that these aren't inert substances, but, indeed, have psychoactive properties that sometimes can interact with other prescribed medications. Please consult with your pharmacists or physician for any multiple or counter reactions of herbs or seasonings, artificial or natural, with prescription or over-the-counter drugs.

Combined with another common phenomenon of home chefferie is a symptom that can occur as easily to home chefs as well as amateur airplane pilots or gymnasts: loss of sense of direction. The construction of an haute cuisine meal—with its many ingredients, steps and timing—requires a whole series of physical maneuvers that could tax the coordination of a well-trained boxer or ballerina. The vegetables in the sauté pan need to be stirred; the Japanese Kobe beef needs to be thinly sliced into a carpaccio; the Caesar salad needs to be mixed; biscuits baking in the oven need to be checked, etc. With or without the complication of alcohol, the home chef can easily lose his or her sense of direction while going through the gymnastic maneuvers that, in a fully equipped commercial restaurant kitchen, would require the talents and aid of several sous chefs.

Symptoms are generally disorientation and inability to tell North from South from East to West in the kitchen. If the chef can't walk a straight line, he knows he's in trouble.

This is why we suggest that every home kitchen, in the medical emergency kit, be provisioned with diphenhydramine, normally employed for motion sickness. A compass and a map of the kitchen could also come in handy.

However, relaxation and deep breathing exercises are the most sensible courses of action for the disoriented home chef. Just take a break!

Two other phenomena can occur in the home kitchen that, if faced unprepared, can cause accidents and damage to the home chef or others. The first is the phenomena of the chef's pants falling down during the acrobatics of meal preparation. Pants can easily drop, as it's sometimes the tendency, in the thrall of unwinding and preparing a grand gourmet meal, to loosen the belt of the trousers. Disaster is definitely on the way should pants fall to the ankles whilst the chef makes his way, with hot pot, pan or plate in hand, between the range or oven, sink and table, or any combination thereof. While any manner of accident can happen, the only prevention for such an occurrence is for chefs to take note and resist the temptation to loosen belts trousers or clothing while in the home kitchen.

The second phenomenon is that of binge eating while cooking. This is a corollary phenomenon to binge drinking while cooking fine cuisine. However, there is no harm in tasting or sampling recipes.

Delusions of grandeur

In the reverie of wonderful aromas, the act of creating a masterpiece and too much wine or booze, mental delusions can descend upon the chef. While chronic mental illness of every stripe and kind can exist outside the home and be brought into the kitchen, we, here, merely want to note that such conditions can occur in the kitchen, amid the euphoria of preparing the meal to beat all meals.

As the chef, for example, goes about his business of slicing truffles or pressing garlic, and quaffing a superb merlot, it's all too easy to slip into delusions of grandeur.

One common delusion that falls upon the home chef is that he should quit his 9-5 daily grind and open a small restaurant in the Berkshires where his culinary art will truly be appreciated. Other delusions can range from the home chef experiencing the uncanny feeling that he is Jesus Christ, or the uncanny feeling that he is NOT Jesus Christ. Or the kitchen changes perspective or appliances begin to take on odd and unusual shapes.

Unless the chef has a chronic mental illness (such as the ongoing, classic delusion that he is the Emperor Napoleon), the only solution to delusions of grandeur or otherwise is to take a break from the kitchen and go do something else. Go lay down for a while, a nap may be in order. And, of course, lay off the vino.

There are other behavioral disorders that can occur, and often do, as the chef works through the hours-long task of meal preparation. One, in particular, results from drinking while cooking. For example, at the exact moment when the white sauce has begun to thicken in the pot and the vegetables in the stir-fry are about to stick in the pan (Sino-French meal), the chef has an extreme urge to urinate. A corollary with this predicament is always that the downstairs bathrooms are/is occupied by family members or guests. And the upstairs bathroom toilet has been clogged for a week, so that's no help.

What to do? What to do? Do we turn down or off the heat and go in search of a spot to obtain immediate relief and thus ruin the meal. Or do we soil our pants?

For the suburban or country chef, this conundrum presents little challenge. The kitchen usually leads to an outdoor patio and the lawn. Relief is but a step away. But what of the chef in a kitchen in a mid-city townhouse or condominium on the 44th floor of an apartment building?

Our advice: Chef, be not proud! Grab any empty container—mixing bowl, large glass measuring cup, cereal or grain container, pot, jar or mug—and let it rip. Better to act like an animal than ruin what otherwise would be a perfectly good recipe. After all, the contents of the container can be disposed of down the sink drain (using all sanitary precautions) and the container washed out.

Preventive measures

- Don't drink too much alcohol while preparing a meal.
- Watch interactions between alcohol and prescription drugs and herbs and seasonings.
- Relax and engage in deep breathing exercises or take a nap if disorientation begins to occur.
- Watch binge eating while preparing meals.
- Don't loosen pants belt while preparing a large meal.

XIV

How To Create a Home Kitchen Medical Emergency Kit

No kitchen should be without these items. Mostly all can be easily obtained over-the-counter at drugstores, pharmacies, or the medicaments section of supermarkets. They should be kept together in a bag or a kit. If a first aid box isn't available, a small tool kit, fishing tackle box, purse or small vinyl or polyethylene bag or knapsack can be used. A label with the words "first-aid kit" should be placed visibly on the outside of the kit. The kit itself should be stored in the kitchen out of the way, in a counter drawer or cabinet, but easily accessible.

1. Long-necked surgical pliers
2. High-intensity flashlight
3. Roll of sterile gauze, or large, sterile gauze pads
4. Tube of antibiotic ointment
5. Tube of cortisone
6. Adhesive bandages, several sizes
7. Moisturizer

8. Sharp scissors or scalpel
9. Anti-flatulent
10. Antacid
11. Pain relievers: ibuprofen or naproxen, and aspirin or acetaminophen
12. Roll of surgical adhesive
13. Cotton balls
14. Sterile gauze pads
15. Thermometer
16. Elastic bandages in several sizes with metal camps
17. Antihistamine, epinephrine
18. Hydrocortisone or diphenhydramine cream
19. Tweezers
20. Ear plugs
21. Rubber tourniquet
22. First-Aid manual
23. Emergency telephone numbers
24. Single-dose injecable hypodermic needle

XV

Kitchen Wall Lists and Diagrams

In this chapter you will find charts and lists that can be posted or kept in a readily-accessible place within the kitchen. (Heimlich diagram is on page 32 and CPR diagram is on page 75)

They are:

1. Medical emergency contact list
2. Map of nearest medical facilities
3. Do's & Don'ts Checklist
4. Common kitchen helpers

Jack Sholl

Medical Emergency Contact List

(Remove page from book by cutting along perforation marks and post in kitchen somewhere near phone.)

General emergencies: 9-1-1

Nearest hospital emergency room: _____

Nearest medical emergency clinic: _____

Family physician: _____

Paramedic service: _____

Police department: _____

Fire department: _____

Poison control center: _____

Others: _____

_____

_____

_____

Map of nearest emergency facilities

(Detach, fill in and place in kitchen)

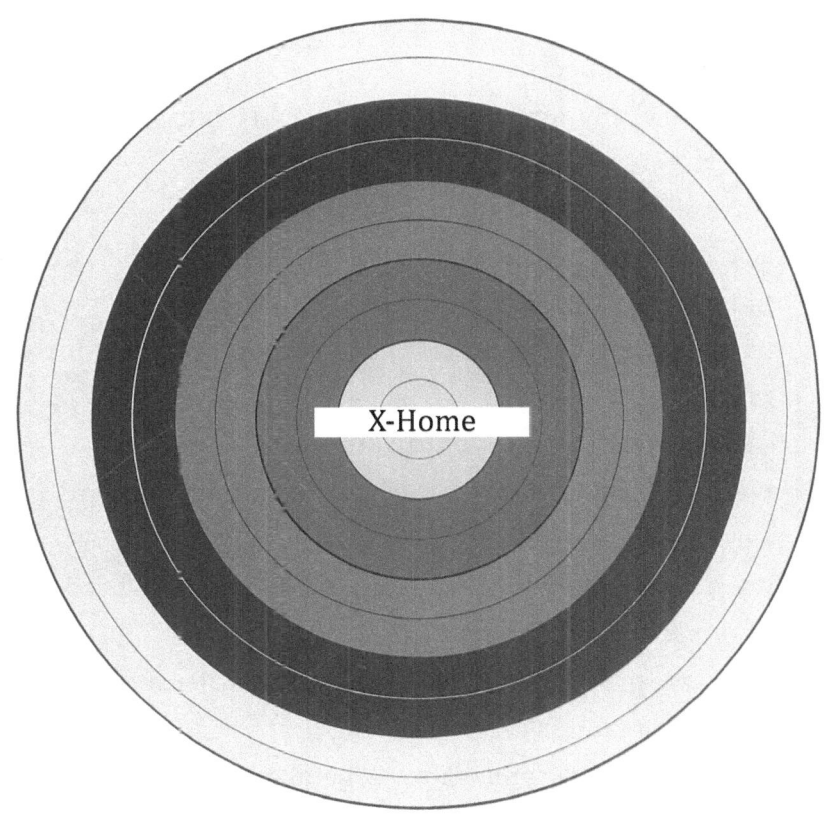

X-Home

Do's and Don'ts

1. Always wear a large full-sized kitchen apron or toque while preparing a meal. Gentlemen, remove your neckties. Ladies, remove your scarves and jewelry.
2. Always use hot pads, preferably gloved hot pads, when handling hot objects.
3. Never poke anything you're holding in your hand with a sharp, pointed utensil.
4. Always slice away from you and take your time.
5. Stack knives and forks downside in the dishwasher, utensil drainer or sink drainer.
6. Throw out anything that comes in contact with broken glass.
7. Slice away from you, never towards you.
8. Never have the knife edge or blade pointed toward you, always away.
9. Always make sure your fingers are sufficiently away from the part or section that's being cut.
10. Always use properly sized knives and utensils, and use them in the right manner.
11. Handle fish bones and spiny vegetables with respect and care.
12. Never take frozen items out of the freezer with wet hands.
13. Use a rubber opener to open tight lids on bottle and jars.
14. When lifting a heavy pot, pan or plate of whole sea bass, hold your arms steady, bend your knees, and lift the assemblage with your knees. Don't try to yank the heavy pot out of the oven with your arms by themselves or your torso.

15. Wear comfortable shoes with non-slip bottoms and good insoles, or sneakers.

16. Don't eat or be observant of how you are eating if you are drunk, inebriated or have had a lot of alcohol.

17. Don't talk or laugh with your mouth stuffed full of food.

18. Make sure you cut your food, particularly hard or firm items, into small or smallish pieces.

19. Be sure to adequately chew the food in your mouth. If you need to make it softer, masticate it with a small sip of water, wine or other beverage.

20. Don't eat rapidly, and certainly don't bolt or wolf down big chunks of food. It's bad for your digestion, it ruins the fine dining experience, and you may choke. Take small mouthfuls of food.

21. Practice the movements of the Heimlich maneuver with a family member or friend to get the feel of it.

22. Use gloves when washing dishes or scouring the countertop with chemical cleaning solutions.

23. Use a good moisturizer on your hands the night before or the morning the day you are cooking.

24. Wash hands thoroughly before and after handling and preparing food.

25. Cook meats, poultry and eggs long enough and at proper heated temperatures to eradicate bacteria.

26. Wash raw vegetables before cooking.

27. Wipe down counters, range, sinks and cutting boards with warm soapy water to eliminate bacteria and cross contamination.

28. Wash all kitchen utensils and serving plates and glasses before using.

29. Disinfect dishrags, dishcloths, sponges and cutting boards in microwave oven.
30. Throw out all spoiled food.
31. Don't let food sit out for a long time in heat before serving to avoid spoilage and contamination.
32. Don't pull away an electrocuted chef from the source of electricity unless you're on an insulated surface.
33. Never use water to put out an electrical fire. Suffocate it or use of a foam fire extinguisher.
34. Be sensitive to lactose intolerance among guests.
35. Be sensitive to the use of beans, sugar, and artificial sweeteners in recipes.
36. Avoid highly acidic food.
37. Have breath mints on hand after dinner.
38. Be especially careful removing heavy objects from overhead cabinets.
39. Clean up spills of water, liquids and slippery vegetables on the floor right away.
40. As with precautions for back injuries, wear shoes with non-slip soles or sneakers.
41. Use non-slip wax on the kitchen floor.
42. Don't drink too much alcohol while preparing a meal.
43. Watch interactions between alcohol and prescription drugs and herbs, and between prescription drugs and herbs and seasonings.
44. Relax and engage in deep breathing exercises, or take a nap if disorientation begins to occur.
45. Watch binge eating while preparing meals.
46. Don't loosen pants belt while preparing a large meal.
47. Have sterile cotton balls or earplugs on hand.

Common kitchen helpers

The following is a small list of items commonly found in the kitchen that may be handy in a medical emergency or medical distress or discomfort

1. Bag of frozen peas
2. Bags of other loose frozen vegetables
3. Ice
4. Pre-filled liquid ice pack
5. Bicarbonate of soda, baking powder
6. Parsley
7. Chamomile, peppermint, anise, catnip or fennel tea
8. Ginger, ginger tea or gingerroot

XVI

Resources

Government:

Centers for Disease Control and Prevention
1600 Clifton Rd.
Atlanta, GA 30333
Tel: (800) 311-3245 www.cdc.gov

U.S. Consumer Product Safety Commission
4330 East-West Highway
Bethesda, MD 20814
Tel: (800) 638-2772 www.cpsc.gov

Department of Health and Human Services
200 Independence Avenue, SW
Washington, DC 20201
Tel: (877) 696-6775 www.hhs.gov

Health Resources and Services Administration
5600 Fishers Lane
Rockville, MD 20857
Tel: (888) 275-4772 www.hrsa.gov

National Library of Medicine
8600 Rockville Pike
Bethesda, MD 20894
Tel: (888) 346-3656 www.nlm.nih.gov

Medical and Other Associations:

American College of Emergency Physicians
1125 Executive Circle
Irving, TX 75038
Tel: (800) 798-1822 www.acep.org

American Council on Science and Health
1995 Broadway, Ste. 202
New York, NY 10023
Tel: (866) 905-2694 www.acsh.org

American Heart Association
7272 Greenville Ave.
Dallas, TX 75231
Tel: (800) 242-8721 www.heart.org

American Hospital Association
155 N. Wacker Dr.
Chicago, Illinois 60606
Tel: (800) 424-4301 www.aha.org

American Medical Association
515 N. State St.
Chicago, IL 60654
Tel: (800) 621-8335 www.ama-assn.org

American Optometric Association
243 N. Lindbergh Blvd.
St. Louis, MO 63141
Tel: (800) 365-2219 www.aoa.org

American Public Health Association
800 I St., NW
Washington, DC 20001
Tel: (202) 777-2742 www.apha.org

American Red Cross
2025 E St.
Washington, DC 20006
Tel: (800) 733-2767 www.redcross.org

American Academy of Dermatology
930 E. Woodfield Rd.
Schaumburg, IL 60173
Tel: (866) 503-7546 www.aad.org

American Society for Dermatologic Surgery
5550 Meadowbrook Dr., Ste. 120
Rolling Meadows, IL 60008
Tel: (708) 330-9830 www.asds.net

American College of Gastroenterology
6400 Goldsboro Rd., Ste. 200
Bethesda, MD 20817
Tel: (301) 263-9000 www.gi.org

American Society for Gastrointestinal Endoscopy
1520 Kensington Rd., Ste. 202
Oak Brook, IL 60523
Tel: (866) 353-2743 www.asge.org

American Head and Neck Society
11300 W. Olympic Blvd., Ste. 600
Los Angeles, CA 90064
Tel: (412) 647-2227 www.ahns.info

American Society for Surgery of the Hand
822 West Washington Blvd.
Chicago, IL, 60607
Tel: (312) 880-1900 www.assh.org

American Society of Colon and Rectal Surgeons
85 West Algonquin Rd., Ste. 550
Arlington Heights, IL 60005
Tel: (847) 290-9184 www.fascrs.org

American Society of Contemporary
Medicine, Surgery and Ophthalmology
820 North Orleans St., Ste. 208
Chicago, IL 60610
Tel: (847) 677-9093 ascmso.accountsupport.com

American Society of Plastic Surgeons
444 East Algonquin Rd.
Arlington Heights, IL 60005
Tel: (847) 228-9900 www.plasticsurgery.org

American Spinal Injury Association
2020 Peachtree Rd., NW
Atlanta, GA 30309
Tel: (404) 355-9772 www.asia-spinalinjury.org

Association of American Physicians and Surgeons
1601 North Tucson Blvd., Ste. 9
Tucson, AZ 85716
Tel: (800) 635-1196 www.aapsonline.org

Bureau of Primary Health Care
5600 Fishers Lane
Rockville, MD 20857
Tel: (888) 275-4772 bphc.hrsa.gov

National Association for Home Care and Hospice
228 Seventh Street, SE
Washington, DC 20003
Tel: (202) 547-7424 www.nahc.org

National Association of Public
Hospitals and Health Systems
1301 Pennsylvania Ave NW, Ste. 950
Washington, DC 20004
Tel: (202) 585-0100 naph@naph.org

National Health Council
1730 M Street, NW, Ste. 500
Washington, DC 20036
Tel: (202) 785-3910 www.nationalhealthcouncil.org

National Medical Association
8403 Colesville Rd., Ste. 920
Silver Spring, MD 20910
Tel: (800) 662-0554 www.nmanet.org

Society for Surgery of the Alimentary Tract
500 Cummings Center, Ste. 4550
Beverly, MA 01915
Tel: (978) 927-8330 www.ssat.com

Society of Thoracic Surgeons
633 North Saint Claire St.
Chicago, IL 60611
Tel: (312) 202-5800 www.sts.org

The Spinal Cord Society
1905 County Highway
1 Fergus Falls, MN 56537
Tel: (218) 739-5252 www.spinalcordsociety.com

American Academy of Dermatology
1445 New York Avenue, NW, Ste. 800
Washington, DC 20005
Tel: (866) 503-7546 www.aad.org

American Academy of Neurology
201 Chicago Ave.
Minneapolis, MN 55415
Tel: (800) 879-1960 www.aan.com

The American Academy of Neurological and Orthopaedic
Surgeons
1516 N. Lakeshore Dr.
Chicago, IL 60610
Tel: (800) 766-3427 www.aanos.org

American Association of Hip and Knee Surgeons
6300 North River Rd., Ste. 615
Rosemont, IL 60018
Tel: (847) 698-1200 www.aahks.org

Association of Orthopaedic Foot and Angle Surgeons
6300 North River Rd.
Rosemont, IL 60018
Tel: (847) 698-4654 www.aofas.org

American Association of Orthopaedic Medicine
600 Pembrook Dr.
Woodland Park, CO 80863
Tel: (888) 687-1920 www.aaomed.org

American College of Occupational and Environmental Medicine
25 Northwest Point Blvd., Ste. 700
Elk Grove Village, IL 60007
Tel: (847) 818-1800 www.acoem.org

American Academy of Ophthalmology
655 Beach St.
San Francisco, CA 94109
Tel: (415) 561-8500 www.aao.org

American Board of Psychiatry and Neurology, Inc.
2150 East Lake Cook Rd., Ste. 900
Buffalo Grove, IL 60089
Tel: (847) 229-6600 www.abpn.com

National Restaurant Association
2055 L Street, NW
Washington, DC 20036
Tel: (800) 424-5156 www.restaurant.org

National Restaurant Association Educational Foundation
175 West Jackson Blvd., Ste. 1500
Chicago, IL 60606
Tel: (800) 765-2122 www.nraef.org

Consumers Union
101 Truman Avenue
Yonkers, NY 10703
Tel: (914) 378-2000 www.consumersunion.org

Centers for Disease Control
1600 Clifton Road
Atlanta, GA 30333
Tel: (404) 639-3311 www.cdc.gov

Food and Drug Administration
10903 New Hampshire Avenue
Silver Spring, MD 20993
Tel: (888) 463-6332 www.fda.gov

XVII

Supplies

CPR Training
> American Heart Association
> 7272 Greenville Ave.
> Dallas, TX 75231
> Tel: (800) 242-8721 www.heart.org

> American Red Cross
> 2025 E St.
> Washington, DC 20006
> Tel: (800) 733-2767 www.redcross.org

Heimlich Training
> American Red Cross
> 2025 E St.
> Washington, DC 20006
> Tel: (800) 733-2767 www.redcross.org

First Aid Posters and Videos

National Restaurant Assn. Educational Foundation

—Workforce Safety Action Kit

—"Preventing Lifting and Carrying Injuries" video

—"Preventing Slips, Trips and Falls" video

National Restaurant Association

2055 L Street, NW

Washington, DC 20036

Tel: (800) 424-5156 www.restaurant.org

XVIII

Further Reading

The American Medical Associations Handbook of First Aid and
  Emergency Care
(Scientifics, www.scientificsonline.com, (800) 818-4955)
Physicians' Desk Reference
Merck Manual
Grey's Anatomy
Boy Scouts of America First Aid Manual

References

Orange County Register (Ca.) Jan. 14, 2000, p. 1 (via Chicago
  Tribune)
Home Safety Network, UK Department of Trade and Industry
Frostbite. McKinley Health Center, University of Illinois at
  Urbana-Champaign, http://www.McKinley.UIUC.edi/health-
  info; Frostbite, C. Crawford Mechem, M.D. http://www.
  emedicine.com/emerg/topic 209.htm

WebMD Medical News, May 22, 2000

Physicians Committee for Responsible Medicine, Foodborne Illness, http://www.PCRM.org/health,Preventive Medicine-Medicine/foodborne-illness.html

Lactose intolerance. Orange County Register (via New York Times), Jan. 14, 2002, p. 9.

Index

Disclaimer Information

As this guide is a common-sense resource stating time-honored applications and uses of commonly available resources, the author and all parties associated with the publication of this work are not responsible nor liable for any diagnosis, medical treatment or the result of any diagnosis or medical treatment relied upon by persons using information contained in this book. As emphasized within the content of this guide, proper medical diagnosis and treatment in emergency and follow-up examination and treatment is solely within the purview of the medical profession and trained medical and paramedical personnel. The authors and all parties associated with the production and publication of this book will not be liable to any reader for any inaccuracies, errors or omissions, regardless of cause, or for any damages (whether direct or indirect, consequential, punitive or exemplary) resulting therefrom, or for any actions taken in reliance upon this work, which has been culled from a number of sources and which may not be inclusive. We make no representations or warranties nor accept liability for performance of any products, procedures or devices in this guide. Any questions pertaining to these products should be directed to the institution or manufacturers providing these entities.

#